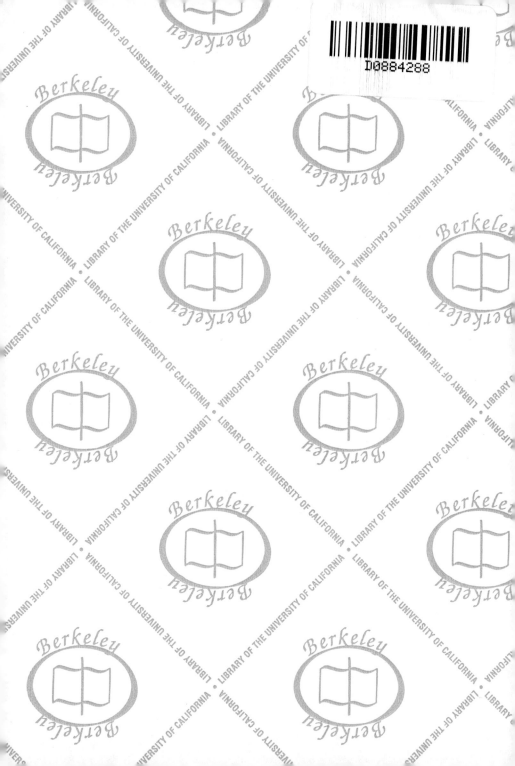

MEDICAL TERMS

THEIR ROOTS AND ORIGINS

MEDICAL TERMS

THEIR ROOTS AND ORIGINS

A.R. TINDALL

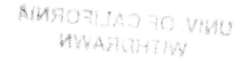

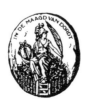

SWETS & ZEITLINGER PUBLISHERS

LISSE ABINGDON EXTON (PA) TOKYO

Library of Congress Cataloging-in-Publication Data

Tindall, A.R. (Alex R.), 1924-
  Medical terms : their roots and origins / A.R. Tindall.
      p.   cm.
  Includes bibliographical references.
  ISBN 9026514980
  1. Medicine--Terminology. 2. English language--Etymology.
1. Title.
  [DNLM: 1. Nomenclature. W 15 T588m 1997]
R123.T56 1997
610'.1'4--DC21
DNLM/DLC
for Library of Congress   97-26853
                                                              CIP

Cover design: Magenta Grafische Produkties, Bert Haagsman
Printed in the Netherlands by Krips, Meppel

ISBN 90 265 14980

Table of Contents

R123
T56
1997
HEAL

Preface

It is no longer the case today that those entering and practising medical sciences are familiar with Latin and Greek, so that much of the terminology is puzzling. This guide is meant to be simple enough to use for those who lack acquaintance with the classical languages. My many years of overseas experience teaching medical students who were not native speakers of English but did use textbooks in English, showed that the terminology seemed without form or pattern to them. It was these students in this situation that persuaded me that this book was needed. With the insight this book gives, almost all medical terminology becomes comprehensible and sensible.

Medical Terms: Their Roots and Origins is not designed for classical scholars. It is for those who are curious about and interested in the origins of one of the most technical and specialised jargons in the world. It is hoped that this book will encourage an interest in the language of the medical sciences which can bring understanding and appreciation of the heritage on which it is built, as well as a greater understanding for the meanings of the terms themselves. At the same time it must be emphasised that this is not a medical dictionary and has quite a different purpose.

The reader is not burdened with details of Latin and Greek declensions. The only criterion used in selecting the forms of the root words listed has been one of utility: will it help readers without knowledge of Greek or Latin to find out and understand the terms they use? For those who do know something of these languages, it is hoped that this book will remind them of the connotations of the words with which they are more or less familiar.

This book aims to give readers access to the information that will enable them to discover the significance of the terms they use. For this reason the Greek words are written in the Latin alphabet – in this way they are easier to understand, although, from the point of view of those familiar with the Greek alphabet this is a pity. Differences between pairs of letters in Greek are lost because they are transliterated by the same letter in Latin and English.

There are three sections to the book. Section 1 lists nearly two thousand word roots in alphabetical order. Each is given first its original meaning, followed by an example taken from medical terminology with its modern meaning, where this differs from the original.

An acquaintance with medical terminology will quickly show that some easily recognised root words occur quite often: *-graph, -gram, cardio-* and *-cephalon*, for instance. Unfortunately, it is not always so simple, and Section 2 is added to show how a selection of medical terms may be subdivided into their constituent parts.

Section 3 is an alphabetical index of words used in English medical terms, with their classical equivalents.

How to use this book
The student may already know the roots from which a medical term is derived and may only wish to find out what the constituent parts meant originally and mean now. In that case only Section 1 is required. For example, *pachyblepharon* is built from two roots: *pachys* and *blepharon*. From Section 1 we find that *pachys* means thick or thickened, while *blepharon* means the eyelid. Thus *pachyblepharon* is used to describe the condition of unusually thick eyelids. Roots words in Greek or Latin may not be spelt quite as in English, but simple inspection will show which roots are the correct ones.

On the other hand, one may be puzzled by a term and cannot be sure from which roots it was constructed. In that case the list in Section 2 should be consulted. Although there are over two thousand terms in this list, it is impossible to include all the medical terms that exist. If the word sought is not listed, a search for similar terms will quickly show how the unlisted term is to be divided and understood. Each constituent part can then be found in Section 1.

It has to be recognised that medical terminology has a long time-span. Coming from ancient Greece, and colonising the Latin of Rome somewhat later, the learning of the ancient world was largely preserved by Arabic scholars during the dark ages. It was translated back into mediaeval Latin at the Renaissance, and since that time many more terms have been needed, and many more root words from Greek and Latin have been taken into use. These new terms were consistent with the older forms in most cases; however, a few mistakes were made and have crept into modern use, for example, the use of the term *diapedesis* instead of *diapeiresis*. The entries in Section 1 make this clear. Also in a few cases, the wrong spelling has been used. This has been corrected nearer to the original, e.g., instead of *orrhorrhoea, ororrhoea* is given since it comes from *oros*. A few words have been left in compound form, because to divide them is to no advantage: e.g., *enchyma, ependyma, diastole,* and a few suffices such as -ia and -ic are not treated separately.

All Latin words have been checked with several dictionaries (see list of references); Greek words have been checked against Liddel and Scott's *Greek-English Lexicon* and the *Shorter Oxford English Dictionary*. It is neither possible nor desirable to give all meanings of many roots: there are 27 entries in the Oxford Latin Dictionary for *cado*, for example.

Of course, thousands of English words are derived more or less directly from the classical languages and one would need a very large book to cover all the root words involved in the origin of the English language. Thus it has been necessary to omit word roots commonly met with in every day English, such as *puncture* (acupuncture), *phase* (telophase) and *-ase* (amylase).

The book relates to the medical and dental sciences only, and does not cover other biological sciences, and for this reason the names of nearly all organisms have been omitted.

Greek words beginning with 'rh...' have '-rrh...', when forming a compound with another word root, e.g., 'rheology' but 'diarrhoea', and this is shown in Section 2. Where a term is written with the letter 'c' today, this has been retained, even though the original spelling used 'k'; for example *cardia, cranion;* but sometimes the 'k' has been kept, as in *kinesis*. In many cases the terms are cross-referenced to avoid uncertainty.

The word *cele* meant originally a tumour or swelling, while *coel-* is derived from *coilos,* meaning hollow. These two roots have been muddled in many terms. It is suggested that *cele* should be used where the swelling is filled with tissue, and *coel* should be applied to hollow swellings.

The diphthongs 'ae' and 'oe' have been kept, e.g., *haemoglobin, aesthesia, oedema*. These are nearer to the classical originals, but in current use, and especially American use, the single letter 'e' is used alone. The distinction can be important. Without a diphthong, *egophony* appears to mean the sound one makes oneself. Spelt correctly, *aegophony*, we see that it comes from *aigos,* and means the sound goats make. Perhaps most would agree it is desirable to differentiate between these two meanings and for the diphthong forms to be retained!

A few word roots have been included which are from other languages, and a very few are of uncertain etymology and are indicated by a question mark. In Section 3 words that have very radically changed from their original meanings are given an asterisk and may be checked in Section 1.

Classicists may be disturbed by what they may see as cavalier treatment in some cases. I can only plead in defence that for those without the advantages of a background in Greek and Latin, it is more important to arouse interest by making the information easily accessible, than to worry too much about the minutiae.

Perhaps we should consider returning to the study of these languages in order to enhance clarity and meaningfulness in the ever-expanding medical terminology. As E.C. Jaeger said in his book *A Source-Book of Biological Names and Terms,* about those who coin new terms "... (they) have proved themselves to be word butchers of the meanest sort...The type of words to which I refer (are) words in which the beautiful classical roots have been chopped into halves, thirds or quarters and combined with other mutilated elements, without following any proper rule of word building. Such practices are inexcusable and should be condemned by all students who have any regard for the ethics and aesthetics of orthography." May those who wish to create a new term accept the guidance of a classical scholar before it is introduced.

It is a pleasure to acknowledge the help given in the preparation of this book by many colleagues and friends, especially Jens Lauesen and Hugh Allen.

Books consulted

A. Medical

Dorland's illustrated medical dictionary. Philadelphia, Saunders, 1981.
Jablonski, S. *The illustrated dictionary of dentistry.* Philadelphia, Saunders, 1982.

B. Languages

Ernout, A. & Meillet, A. *Dictionaire etymologique de la langue latine.* Paris, Librarie Klincksieck, 1967. 4th edition.
Du Cange. *Glossorum mediae et infimae latinitatis.* Paris, Librarie des Sciences et des Arts, 1937.
Souter, A. *Glossary of later Latin to 600 AD.* Oxford, Clarendon Press, 1964.
Smyth, H.W. *Greek grammar.* Cambridge, MA, Harvard University Press, 1974.
Simpson, D.P. *Latin-English, English-Latin dictionary.* London, Casssel, 1979.
Morland, H. *Latinsk ordbok.* Oslo, Cappellen, 1965.
Liddell & Scott. *Greek-English Lexicon.* Oxford, Clarendon Press, 1968.
Oxford Latin dictionary. Oxford, Clarendon Press, 1968-1985.
Shorter Oxford English dictionary. Oxford, Clarendon Press, 1965

C. Terminology

Bentz, G. *Latin for medicinare.* Lund, Gleerup, 1972.
Field, E.J. & Harrison, R.J. *Anatomical terms: their origin and derivation.* Cambridge, Heffer, 1947
Jaeger, E.C. *A source-book of biological names and terms.* Springfield IL, Charles C. Thomas, 1955.
Patterson, S.R. & Thompson, L.S. *Medical terminology from Greek and Latin.* Troy N.Y., Whitston, 1978.
Pepper, O.H.P. *Medical etymology.* Philadelphia, Saunders, 1949.
Roberts, F. *Medical terms: their origin and construction.* London, Heinemann Medical Books, 1971.

Skinner, H.A. *The origin of medical terms.* Baltimore, Williams and Wilkins, 1961.

Sorensen, E. & Nielsen, E.H. *Terminologica medicina.* Copenhagen, Arnold Busck, 1961.

Abbreviations

A	Arabic
D	German
F	French
G	Greek
I	Italian
L	Latin

cf.	compare
comp.	comparative
dim.	diminutive
fut.	future
gen.	genitive
plur.	plural
q.v.	which may be looked at
sup.	superlative

Section 1

Latin and Greek word-roots used in medical terminology

"The question is", said Alice,
"whether you can make words mean so many different things."

Lewis Carroll – '*Alice through the looking glass.*'

A

a, ab	L	Movement away from. ABDUCT – to move a part of the body away from the mid-line.
a, an	G	A negation or absence of something. ACAPNIA – an absence of carbon dioxide, often used improperly for reduced carbon dioxide concentration. See **capnos**
ab		See **a.**
ablatus	L	Removed. ABLATION – extirpation of a part.
abluo; ablutum	L	To wash away; washed clean. ABLUTION – washing or cleansing with water. See also **luo.**
abortus	L	Prematurely born, miscarried. ABORTUS – a small foetus which cannot survive.
abscessus	L	Abscess, congestion. ABSCESS.
ac		See **a.**
acantha	G	A thorn, spine, spike. ACANTHOLYSIS – the breaking of the intercellular connections between the prickle-cells of the epidermis.
acari	G	Tiny, something very small. ACARIASIS – infected with mites.
Acarus		A kind of mite. See **acari.**
acervus	L	A heap. ACERVULUS – a later modification, now used to mean gritty material lying in association with the choroid plexus of the brain.
acesis	G	A cure, healing, repair. ACESODYNE – relieving pain.
acetabulum	L	A (vinegar) cup, cup-shaped structures, the socket of the hip-joint. ACETABULUM – the articular cup for the femoral head. Cf. cotyloid.
acetum	L	Acid, vinegar. ACETONAEMIA – with excess ketones in the blood. See also **keto.**
achne	G	Froth, chaff, down on a surface, loose surface material. ACNE – an inflammation of the skin. Some believe this word to come from **acme.**
acinus	L	A grape, berry, shaped so. ACINI – subdivisions of a gland shaped like a multilocular berry.
acme	G	A point, edge, eruption on the face. ACMAESTHESIA – the feeling of a sharp point.
acne		See **achne, acme.**

aco		See **acos.**
acon	G	Involuntary, constrained, unwilling. ACONURESIS – involuntary loss of urine.
aconiton	G	*Aconitum anthora* and *A. napellus*. ACONITUM – poisonous plant, source of aconite.
acos	G	A cure, relief, remedy. ACOSGNOSIS – a study of cures.
acouo	G	To hear, listen to. ACOUSTIC – concerned with hearing.
acros	G	An extremity, summit. ACROPHOBIA – a fear of heights.
actin		See **actis** or **actus.**
actis	G	A ray, beam; radially arranged structures. ACTINOMYCETES – fungi with spores in radiating rows.
actus	L	Motion, movement, action. ACTIN – a filamentous protein, involved, with myosin, in muscle contraction.
acumen	L	A sharp point. ACUMINATE – having a sharp point.
acus	L	1. A needle. ACUSTENACULUM – a needle holder. 2. See **acouo.**
ad	L	Towards. ADDUCT – to move a part towards the mid-line. [The "d" becomes "c", "f", "g", "p", "s" or "t" before words beginning with these letters.]
ad	G	1. Derived from - **as** in words such as trias, tetras. Now used as a collective suffix, e.g., TRIAD – a collection of three. 2. Towards the thing given by the main word, e.g., CAUDAD – towards the tail.
adamas	G	Unconquerable; hard steel. ADAMANTINE – pertaining to tooth enamel.
adelphos	G	One of brothers, sons of the same mother. SYNADELPHUS – a conjoined foetal monster. See also **delphys.**
aden	G	A gland. ADENOMA – a tumour with glandular cells.
adeps, adipis	L	Fat. ADIPOSE – tissue with a large fat content. See also **aleipho.**

adipis		See **adeps**.
aditus	L	An entrance, access. ADITUS orbitae – the aperture between the orbit and the cranium.
adjuvans	L	Aiding. ADJUVANT – something assisting or enhancing the effect of treatment, especially in immunology.
adnexus	L	A connexion, a binding (together). ADNEXA – adjuncts of an organ.
advenio	L	To approach, to come from a strange place. ADVENTITIA – external covering layer, especially of blood vessels.
aecon		See **acon**
aego		See **aix**.
aema		See **haima**.
aer	G	Mist, air, gas. AEROBIC – using oxidative metabolism.
aesthesia		See **aisthesis**.
aestivus	L	Summer. AESTIVATION – summer hibernation.
aetio		See **aitia**.
af		See **ad**.
affero	L	To convey, bring towards. AFFERENT – centripetal; opposite to efferent. (See **effero**).
ag		See **ad**. AGGLUTINATE – to collect together.
ago	G	To carry (away), lead towards. See **agogos**.
agogos	G	Leading, drawing forth, eliciting. CHOLEAGOGUE, CHOLAGOGUE – provoking the flow of bile.
agon; agonistes	G	A gathering, place of struggle; contestant. AGONIST – a muscle, opposed by another, the antagonist. Also a drug whose effect in the body is inhibited or opposed by another drug, the antagonist.
agora	G	An assembly place, forum, an open area. AGORAPHOBIA – a fear of open places.
agra		See **agreo**.
agreo	G	To take, seize, catch. Now pain. PODAGRA – the pain of gout in the foot.
ailouros	G	A cat. **Aelurophilia** – an excessive love of cats.
airesis	G	A taking, choice. Now also a drawing together or

		condensation. SYNAERESIS – shrinkage of a gel or blood clot, with extrusion of liquid.
aisthesis	G	Sensation, sensory perception. ANAESTHESIA – without conscious sensation.
aitia	G	Responsibility, blame for, cause. AETIOLOGY – the study of disease causation.
aix, aigos	G	A she-goat. AEGOBRONCHOPHONIA – an unusual bleating sound in the lungs when compressed by a pleural effusion.
akousis		See acouo.
al		See alaos. Also an English adjectival suffix. PLEURAL.
ala	L	A wing. ALA NASI – the outer sides of the nostrils.
alaos	G	Blind. NYCTALOPIA – poor vision at night or in dim light.
alapazo	G	To plunder, empty, carry off. LITHOLAPAXY – crushing a stone in the bladder and washing out the fragments afterwards.
albus; album	L	White; white colour. ALBUMEN – the protein of egg white.
aleipho	G	To anoint with oil, polish. IATRALIPTIC – pertaining to treatment by friction and the rubbing on of oils.
aleteria	G	Wandering, roaming. ALEOCYTE – a wandering cell.
alexo	G	To ward off, defend. ALEXIPYRETIC – hindering fever.
algesis	G	The sense of pain. ALGESIA – sensitivity to pain.
algor	L	Coldness. ALGOR MORTIS – loss of heat from the body after death.
algos	G	Pain, grief. ALGOMETER – an instrument for measuring sensitivity to painful stimuli.
aliptic		See aleipho.
all		See allos.
allache	G	Elsewhere, in another place. ALLACHAESTHESIA – a visual illusion such that things are seen in a wrong position.
allas, allantoin	G	A sausage, a little sausage. ALLANTIASIS – botulism from sausages.

allasso	G	To change, interchange, barter. ALLAXIS – transformation.
allaxis		See **allasso**.
allelon	G	Of one another, mutually, reciprocally. ALLELOMORPH – characteristics which are inherited after Mendelian laws, and the gene pairs responsible for such characters.
allos	G	Other, different. ALLERGY – excessive sensitivity to some substance, often arising from previous contact with the causal agent.
allotrios	G	Alien, not belonging, strange. ALLOTRIOGEUSTIA – an abnormal sense of taste.
alopex; alopecia	G	The fox, mange; bald patches. ALOPECIA – patchy loss of hair.
altrix, altricis	L	A nurse, foster mother. ALTRICIOUS – needing a long period of nursing.
alveus	L	A channel, cavity. ALVEOLAR – having hollows, sacculate.
amauros	G	Dimly seen, obscure, blind. AMAUROSIS – blindness from dysfunction of the nervous system.
amblys	G	Blunt, dull, dim, poorness of vision. AMBLYOPIA – poor vision without lesion of the eye.
ambo	L	On both sides. AMBIDEXTROUS – able to use both hands skilfully. See also **amphi**.
ambulo	L	To walk about. AMBULATORY – able to walk.
amel	F	Enamel. AMELOBLAST – a cell which helps to form tooth enamel.
amnion	G	The caul or membrane around a foetus. AMNIOTIC – pertaining to the foetal membrane, the amnion.
amoeba		See **amoibe**.
amoibe	G	A change, alteration. AMOEBOID – with a changing form.
amphi; ampho	G	Doubly, around, on both sides; both. AMPHICOE LOUS – having two concavities.
amphoteros	G	Pertaining to both of a pair. AMPHOTERIC – substances having both acidic and basic properties and affinities.
amygdale	G	An almond, shaped to. AMYGDALA – an almond-

		shaped structure, e.g., in the fore-brain. Also a tonsil.
amylon	G	Starch. AMYLOIDOSIS – a disease in which a complex of glycoprotein accumulates in various body tissues.
an(a)	G	Upon, increasing, upwards. ANAPHYLAXIS – an unusual or increasing reaction to a foreign substance.
anachoresis	G	A retreat, withdrawal. ANACHORESIS – a sequestering of foreign matter into particular parts of the body.
ancon	G	The elbow. ANCONAD – towards the elbow.
ancylo		See ankylos.
andro		See aner.
aner, andros	G	A man, pertaining to a man. ANDROGEN – a masculizing substance.
angeion	G	A vessel, receptacle. ANGIOGRAM – an X-ray photograph showing the blood vessels.
ankylos	G	Bent, curved, crooked. ANKYLOSTOMA – a parasitic worm with hooks around its mouth.
ankylosis	G	Stiffening of the joints. ANKYLOSIS – stiffening or immobility of joint articulations, due to disease or surgery.
ansa	L	A loop-shaped handle. ANSA – loop-shaped.
anserinus	L	Belonging to a goose. PES ANSERINUS – a structure shaped like a goose-foot, e.g., certain thigh muscles.
ante	L	Before, in time or place. ANTENATAL – before birth.
antheo	G	To burst into bloom, flower, flourish. Now to erupt. EXANTHEM – eruptive fever.
anthrax	G	Coal, carbon, carbuncle (a red semi-precious stone). ANTHRAX – a bacterial disease in which carbuncles or ulcers are common. Possible so named because of the black crust which forms over the ulcerations.
anthropos	G	Humanity. ANTHROPOLOGY – the study of mankind.
ant, anti	G	Against, opposite to. ANTISEPTIC – preventing sepsis.

antron	G	A cave, an inner chamber or place. ANTRUM – a cavity, especially in bones.
ap		See **ad** or **apo**.
aperio	L	To reveal, disclose, open. APERIENT – a laxative or mild purgative.
aph, aphia		See **haphe** or **hapto**.
aphaireo	G	To take from, separate, set aside. PLASMAPHAERESIS – centrifugal separation of blood, and reinjection of the cells.
aphtha	G	"Thrush" in the mouth. APHTHAE – thrush spots, small ulcers in the mouth.
ap(o)	G	From, away from. APOPHYSIS – an outgrowth.
apoplecticos	G	Paralysed. MYELAPOPLEXY – haemorrhage into the spinal cord, resulting in paralysis. See also **plesso**.
appendix	L	An appendage, additional part. APPENDIX.
apsis		See **hapsis**.
arachne	G	Spider's web, thin lines. ARACHNOID membrane – web-like membrane between the meninges, dura mater and pia mater.
arceo	G	To ward off, defend, suffice. AUTARCESIS – natural resistance to infection.
arcesis	G	Aid, service. See **arceo**.
arche	G	Beginning, origin. ARCHENTERON – the primitive, embryonic gut.
arcus	L	A bow, arch. ARCUATE – of curved outline.
argyros	G	Silver. ARGYROPHIL – staining readily with silver.
aristeuo	G	To be best or bravest. ARISTOGENICS – supposed improvement of a race by selective mating of its members.
arkys	G	A net. ARKYOCHROME – a cell with a stainable reticular structure.
arrhenicos	G	Male, masculine. ARRHENOBLASTOMA – an ovarian tumour often causing virilization.
arteria	G	The wind-pipe; later an artery. ARTERY.
arthriticos	G	Gout, arthritic joints. ARTHRITIS.
arthron	G	A joint, especially the ankle. ARTHRITIS – rheumatism of the joints.

arthroo	G	To join together, to articulate (words). DYSARTHRIA – unclear speech or articulation.
articularis	L	Concerned with joints. ARTICULATION – a joining, usually between two bones, with or without the possibility of movement.
aryter, arytaina	G	A cup, jug, ladle. ARYTENOID – shaped like a jug, especially one of the laryngeal cartilages.
as		See **ad.**
ascaris	G	An intestinal worm. ASCARIASIS – infected with Ascaris.
ascos	G	A leather bag, wine-skin or paunch. ASCITES – fluid in the abdomen.
asis		See **iasis** or **osis.**
asper	L	Rough. LINEA ASPERA – rough ridges on the femur for muscle attachment.
aster		See **astron.**
asthma	G	Panting, difficult breathing. ASTHMA.
astragalos	G	One of the vertebrae, the ball of the ankle joint, any small rounded object suitable for playing dice. ASTRAGULUS – the talus bone, articulating with the tibia and fibula.
astron	G	A star. ASTROCYTOMA – a tumour of astrocytes, neuroglial cells with long processes.
at		See **ad.**
atavi	L	Ancestors, especially those of several generations previously. ATAVISTIC – characteristics inherited from remote ancestors.
ateles	G	Unending, imperfect, unaccomplished. ATELECTASIS – incomplete expansion of the lungs after birth; collapse of a lung.
athare	G	Groats, small grains, porridge. ATHEROMA – a mass of degenerate cells within an artery affected by atherosclerosis. Also a sebaceous cyst.
athetos	G	Without position or place, lawless, incompetent. ATHETOSIS – involuntary, incessant movements, especially of the hands.
atopos	G	Strange, paradoxical, unnatural. ATOPY – an inherited disposition to one or other allergic reaction.

atrium	L	An entrance room. ATRIUM – a small chamber.
audio	L	To hear. AUDIOMETRY – measurement of hearing.
auris, auricula	L	The ear, the lobe of the ear. AURINASAL – concerned with the ear and nose.
ausculto	L	To listen attentively. AUSCULTATION – listening to the sounds made by the internal organs of the body.
autos	G	Self. AUTOIMMUNE – reacting against the body's own tissues.
auxe, auxano	G	To increase, aggrandise, grow. ONYCHAUXIS – overgrowth of the nails.
axia, axios	G	Worth, value. CHRONAXIE – the minimum duration of current flow which will provoke a response in a nerve, given twice the rheobase voltage.
axon	G	An axle, axis. AXON – the efferent process of a nerve cell.

B

ba		See **baino** and **batos.**
bacillum	L	A small staff or rod. BACILLUS – a genus of bacteria, but also loosely for any bacteria-like microorganism.
bactron, bacteria	G	A stick, a small staff or rod. BACTERIA – microorganisms multiplying by fission and possessing a cell wall.
baino	G	To go, walk, stand. HYPNOBATIA – somnambulism.
balanos	G	An acorn, shaped so. BALANITIS – inflammation of the glans penis.
ballo	G	To throw, smite. CATABOLISM – breakdown processes in metabolism.
balneum	L	A bathing place. BALNEOTHERAPY – treament by bathing.
baros, barys	G	Weight, heaviness, abundance. HYPERBARIC – applied to gases under greater than normal pressure; also to liquids with a specific gravity greater than a reference liquid, usually water.

basilicos	G	Royal, i.e., important, prominent. BASILAR ARTERY – the main artery in the head.
basis	G	1. Base, foundation. BASOPHIL – having affinity with basic substances. 2. A stepping, step. ABASIA – inability to walk. See **baino**.
bathmos	G	Step, threshold, interval. BATHMOTROPIC – affecting the response threshold of an excitable tissue, either negatively or positively.
bathos	G	Depth. BATHOMORPHIC – having myopia, owing to the eyes being too deep from anterior to posterior.
bathys	G	Deep, copious, profound. BATHYANAESTHESIA – loss of deep sensibility.
batos	G	Passable, accessible. Connected with **baino**, q.v. DIABETIC – with a large excretion of urine and commensurate thirst.
be		See **bios**.
benignus	L	Kind, pleasing. BENIGN tumour – a non-malignant growth.
betic		See **batos**.
bi		See **bis**.
bilis	L	1. Bile. BILIRUBIN – a bile pigment resulting from red cell destruction. 2. See **ilis**.
bios	G	Mode of life, manner of living. BIOLOGY.
bis	L	Twice, double, two. BICEPS – having two heads.
blapto	G	To disable, distract, harm, hurt. IDIOBLAPSIS – a kind of food allergy.
blastos	G	A bud, shoot, embryo, offspring. CHONDROBLAST – a cell which produces cartilage.
blenna	G	Mucus. BLENNORRHEA – a mucous discharge.
blepharon	G	The eyelid. BLEPHAROPTOSIS – drooping of the eyelid.
blepo	G	To look, see, have sight, look towards. HEMIABLEPSIA – poor vision in half of the visual field.
bole	G	A throw, strike, touch. METABOLIC – concerned with the chemical processes of the body.

bolus	L	A throw; a good haul from throwing a fishing net. BOLUS – a mass or lump.
botulus	L	A sausage. BOTULISM – a disease caused by *Clostridium botulinum* often from improperly cooked food.
boubon	G	The groin, a gland (of the groin). BUBONALGIA – pain in the groin.
boule	G	Will, determination. ABOULIA – loss or reduction of will-power or initiative.
bounos	G	A hill, mound. BUNODONT – applied to a tooth with rounded cusps.
bous	G	An ox. BULIMY – abnormal excessive eating.
brachion	G	The arm. BRACHIAL – pertaining to the fore-limb.
brachys	G	Short (in space or time). BRACHYCEPHALIC – with a short, wide head.
bradys	G	Slow, tardy, sluggish. BRADYCARDIA – abnormally low heart rate.
branchion	G	A fin, gill. BRANCHIAL – of the gill region and its homologues.
bregma	G	The front part of the head, the forehead; but also the parietal bones. BREGMA – the intersection of the coronal and sagittal sutures of the skull.
broma	G	Food, meat. BROMATOTOXINS – poisons formed in rotting food.
bromos	G	A foul smell. BROMHIDROSIS – stinking sweat.
bronchos	G	The windpipe. BRONCHIAL – concerned with the lower air passages.
brux		See **brycho**.
bryc(h)o, bryxo	G	To eat noisily, to gnash the teeth. BRUXISM – the grinding of the teeth especially when asleep.
bryo	G	To swell, be full of, to teem with something. EMBRYO.
bu		See **bous**.
bucca	L	The cheek. BUCCAL – pertaining to the cheek.
buc(c)inator	L	A trumpeter. BUCCINATOR – cheek muscle used in blowing.
bulla	L	A boss, bubble, round swelling. BULLA TYMPANI – the bony chamber enclosing the middle ear.

bursa	G	Hide, leather; a pouch made of skin. BURSITIS – inflammation of a bursa.
byssos	G	Threads of flax; linen. BYSSINOSIS – inflammation of the lungs from inhalation of fine threads or particles of cloth.

C

cac		See **cacos**. CACHEXIA – chronic malnutrition and very poor health.
cacos	G	Bad, evil. CACOGENESIS – defective development.
cadaver		See **cado**.
cado; cecidi	L	To fall, slip; dropped. DECIDUA – the tissue lost from the uterus after parturition.
caducous		See **cado**.
caecus	L	Blind. CAECUM – a blind-ending structure.
caedo; cecidi	L	To cut, kill; killed. HOMICIDE – killing a human being.
cainos	G	New, fresh, novel. CAENOGENESIS – the appearance of new ontogenetic features.
caio	G	To burn, set on fire, cauterize. LIPOCAIC – of a substance which hinders the deposition of fat in the liver.
calamos	G	A reed (used to make pens amongst other things), shaped so. CALAMUS SCRIPTORIUS – the floor of the fourth ventricle, said to resemble a pen.
calcar	L	A spur. CALCARINE SULCUS – separates the cuneus and lingual gyri of the occipital lobe.
calcitro	L	To kick, to resist obstinately. RECALCITRANT – refractory, not responding to treatment.
calculus	L	A small stone or pebble; gravel. CALCULUS – a concretion or stone.
calix, calices		See **calyx**.
callosus; callum	L	Having a hard skin; hard, tough skin. CALLUS – a hard patch of horny skin.
calos	G	Beautiful, fair. CALISTHENICS – exercises for grace and strength

calx; calcis	L	1. The heel. CALCANEUS – the bone of the heel. 2. A stone. CALCIPEXY – sequestering of calcium compounds in the body.
calyx	G	The cup-shaped calyx of a flower. CALYX – a cavity of this kind.
campto	G	To bend, bow down, turn around. ACAMPSIA – rigidity, especially of a joint.
canaliculus	L	A small canal. CANALICULUS.
cancer	L	A crab. CANCER – malignant tumour. See also **carcinos.**
candidus	L	Shining white, glistening. CANDIDA – a fungus affecting mucous membranes and skin, and forming white spots.
canthos	G	The metal tyre on a wooden wheel, later applied to the rim of the eyelid, and then the corner of the eye. CANTHUS – the outer or inner corner of the eye, between the two eyelids.
capio	L	To take, seize, receive. RECEPTOR – a structure in the body which responds specifically to changes which impinge upon it.
capitis		See **caput.**
capnos	G	Smoke, vapour. HYPERCAPNIA – having a higher than normal tension of carbon dioxide in the blood.
capsa; capsula	L	A circular box for books; a small chest. ENCAPSULATE – to enclose in a sac-like structure.
caput, capitis	L	The head, the chief part. BICEPS – a muscle with two heads or origins. See also **cephale.**
carbo	L	Coal, charcoal; carbonaceous. CARBOHYDRATE – one of the three main types of food.
carcinos	G	A crab; a cancre or ulcer; pincers. CARCINOMA – disease due to a malignant, gripping tumour.
cardia	G	The heart. CARDIECTASIS – dilation of the heart.
caries	L	Rottenness, decay. CARIES.
carina	L	A keel of a ship, shaped so. CARINATE – having a keel, or keel-like.
caro; carnis	L	The body (not the mind); of the flesh. CARNEOUS – fleshy.

caros	G	Heavy drowsiness, sleep. CAROTID – an artery to the brain. (It was believed that pressure on this vessel would induce torpor!)
carpos	G	The wrist. CARPOMETACARPAL – applied to the articulation between the wrist and the bones of the hand.
cary		See **karyon.**
caseus	L	Cheese. CASEOSERUM – an antiserum produced by immunisation with casein.
cat(a)	G	Downwards, negative. CATABOLISM – metabolic breakdown.
catarrh		See **cata** and **rheo.**
catarxis	G	A beginning. PROCATARXIS – a predisposition to a disease.
catharsis	G	A cleansing, purgation. CATHARSIS – a cleansing or purgation of either the body, or the mind.
catheter	G	An instrument for emptying the bladder; something inserted; a pessary. CATHETER – a flexible tube inserted to remove fluid from, or to introduce fluid into, the body.
cathexis	G	Retention, holding, possession. ACATHEXIA – inability to retain secretions in the body.
cathisis	G	Sitting, sitting down. ACATHISIA – inability to sit quietly, restlessness.
cauda	L	The tail. CAUDAL – concerned with the tail.
causos	G	Heat, fever, heartburn. CAUSALGIA – a persistent burning pain after peripheral nerve injury.
causticos	G	Caustic, corrosive. CAUSTIC.
cauterion	G	Branding iron. CAUTERY – an instrument for destroying tissue by a caustic substance or by burning.
cele	G	A tumour, swelling. VARICOCELE – swollen pampiniform blood vessels forming a swelling in the scrotum. See also **kele.**
celero	L	To hasten, to accelerate. PULSUS CELER – a fast pulse.
cen		See **coinos** or **cainos** or **cenos.**
cenos	G	Empty, void. HYDROCENOSIS – removal of fluid.

centeo	G	To prick, sting. AMNIOCENTESIS – removal of some amniotic fluid by abdominal puncture.
cephale	G	The head. CEPHALIC – pertaining to the head.
ceps		See caput.
cept		See concipio or recipio or capio.
cera; cereus	L	Wax; waxen. CERUMEN – ear wax. See also keras.
ceras		See keras.
cercos	G	A tail. CERCOMONAS – a protozoon with two tails, sometimes found in humans.
cerebellum	L	A little brain. CEREBELLUM.
cerebrum	L	The brain. CEREBRUM – the cerebral hemispheres.
cereolus		See cera.
cervix; cervicis	L	The neck; of it. CERVICAL – appertaining to a neck.
chaite	G	Hair, a mane, helmet crest. SPIROCHAETA – a bacterium of twisted shape and with hair-like filaments.
chalao	G	To relax, loosen, let go, yield. CHALASIA – relaxation, especially of an opening.
chalazao	G	To hail; to be afflicted with pimples. CHALAZION – a cyst of a meibomian gland on the eyelid.
chancre		See carcinos. CHANCRE – a venereal ulcer.
chasma	G	A large gap, gulf. CHASMA – an opening, a wide gap.
cheilos	G	A lip, brim. CHEILITIS – inflammation of the lips.
cheir	G	The hand. CHIROPODIST – one treating the foot, originally by manipulation, i.e., using the hands. Cf. podiatrist.
chele		See cele.
cheme	G	Gaping, yawning, a clam. See chemosis.
chemosis	G	An affliction of the cornea which swells and looks like a cockle-shell. CHEMOSIS – excessive oedema between the conjuctiva and cornea. See cheme.
cheo	G	To pour, shed, liquify, dissolve. SYNCHYSIS – liquifaction of the vitreous humour.
chezo	G	To defaecate, go to stool. HAEMATOCHEZIA – bloody faeces.
chiasma	G	A crossing over, from the letter chi, X. CHIASM.
chimaira	G	A female goat; a mythical monster. CHIMAERA –

an organism derived from the cells of more than one zygote. Sometimes spelled chimera.

chilo   See **cheilos.**

chir   See **cheir.**

chlamys   G   A short cloak. BALANOCHLAMYDITIS – inflammation of the glans clitoridis and its hood.

chloazo   G   To be bright green. CHLOASMA – various yellowish-brown discolorations on the skin; melasma.

chloros   G   Green, yellowish, pale. ACHLOROPSIA – inability to see green.

chole   G   Bile. DUCTUS CHOLEDOCHUS – the (common) bile duct.

cholin   See **chole.**

chondros   G   1. A grain. MITOCHONDRIA – small cytoplasmic organelles.

2. Gristle, cartilage, especially that attaching the ribs to the sternum. HYPOCHONDRIUM – the region just below the diaphragm with the spleen supposed to be the site of morbid anxiety about one's health.

chorde   G   Guts, a string made from gut. NOTOCHORD – the embryological dorsal midline structure lying adjacent to the neural tube in chordates.

choreia   G   A choral dance. CHOREA – continuous, jerky, involuntary movements.

chorion   G   A foetal membrane, afterbirth; intestinal membranes. CHORION – the foetal component of the developing placenta, with villi and rich vascularisation.

chrestos   G   Useful, serviceable. ACHRESTIC – pertaining to something present but not used in the processes of the body.

chroma   G   The skin, complexion, colour. CHROMOSOME – one of the hereditary units of DNA in the nucleus which can be stained at certain phases of cell division. See also **chros.**

chronos   G   Time. CHRONIS – long lasting.

chros, chrotos	G	The body surface, the skin, its colour. CHROTOPLAST – a skin cell. See also **chroma**.
chrysos	G	Gold, its colour. CHRYSODERMA- gold deposited in the skin.
chthlon	G	The earth, world, ground. NOSOCHTHONOGRAPHY – the mapping of epidemics and other diseases.
chylos	G	Juice. CHYLE – the fluid in the lacteals in the villi.
chy, chym	G	1. See **cheo**. ECCHYMOSIS – a skin haemorrhage giving a bluish patch. 2. See **enchyma**.
chymos	G	A fluid, that which flows. CHYME, CHYMUS – the semi-fluid material in the gut.
chysis	G	A pouring forth; melting and casting; a flood. CIRSENCHYSIS – injecting a sclerosing substance into varicose veins.
cicatrix	L	A scar. CICATRIX.
cid, cido		See **caedo** or **cado**.
cilium	L	An eye-lid or eye-lash. CILIA – motile, hair-like organelles.
cineris		See **cinis**.
cingulum	L	A girdle. CINGULUM – an encircling structure, especially that around the corpus callosum.
cinis	L	Ashes. CINERA – grey matter of the central nervous system (the colour of ashes).
cion	G	A pillar, column, the nasal septum, the uvula. CIONITIS – inflammation of the uvula. See **kion**.
cirrhos		See **cirros**.
cirros	G	Yellowish-brown. CIRRHOSIS – liver disease, often showing as jaundice.
cirsos	G	A varicocoel, a varicosed vein. CIRSENCHYSIS – varicose vein injection. Cf. varix.
cision		See **caedo**.
clados	G	A branch; of a tree or a blood vessel. NEUROCLADISM – the sprouting of new growth from the ends of sectioned nerves.
clao; clasis	G	To break, break off; fracture. OSTEOCLAST – a cell concerned with breakdown of bone.

clasma	G	A fragment, moiety, piece. CLASMATOCYTE – a cell from which a part breaks of the secretory process.
clast		See clao.
claudico	L	To limp, be lame, be defective. CLAUDICATION – debilitating pain on walking.
claudo	L	To enclose, shut away. See claustrum.
claustrum	L	A means of confinement. CLAUSTROPHOBIA – dread of confinement or being in an enclosed place.
clavis	L	A key, shaped so. CLAVICLE – the bone between the sternum and the scapula. See also cleis.
clavus	L	A (metal) nail. CLAVUS – a horny skin growth.
cleis; cleidosis	G	1. A bolt, hook, fastening, key; the collar bone. CLEIDOCOSTAL – concerned with the clavicle and ribs. 2. See kleio.
cleitoris	G	The clitoris. CLITORIS.
climacter	G	A rung of a ladder, a special event in one's life. CLIMACTERIC – changes accompanying the menopause in normal women.
cline	G	A couch, bed. CLINICAL – directly concerned with sicknesses and their treatment. See also clino.
clinicos	G	Applied to a physician who sees patients in bed. CLINICIAN – See also cline and clino.
clino	G	To incline, bend, lean upon. CLINOMETER – a device to measure angular movements, especially ocular. See also cline.
clitic		See clino. ANACLITIC – using another in psychological support, especially of a child and its parents.
clitoris		See cleitoris.
clivus	L	A slope, elevation. CLIVUS – a part of the skull sloping upwards from the foramen magnum.
clonos	G	Agitated movements. turmoil. CLONUS – rapid, abnormal, reflex movements.
clunis	L	The buttocks. CLUNEAL – pertaining to the buttocks.
clyster	G	A clyster syringe, an enema. ENTEROCLYSIS – pas-

		sage of nutrient liquid into the gut, by means of a catheter.
cneme	G	The leg, tibia. GASTROCNEMIUS – a large muscle at the back of the leg.
coarcto		See **coarto**.
coarto	L	To draw together, compress, shorten. COARTATION – constriction of a vessel. Sometimes misspelled coarctation.
coccos	G	A grain, seed, pill. COCCAL bacteria – small spheroidal bacteria.
coccyx	G	A cuckoo. COCCYX – the inferior vertebrae of the spine.
cochlarion	G	A spoon in the form of a snail shell. COC(H)LEARE – a spoon.
cochlias	G	A snail, spirally twisted. COCHLEA the spirally shaped inner ear.
coel		See **coilos, coilia**.
coeno		See **coinos**.
coilia	G	The abdomen, with or without the thorax; any body cavity. COELOME – the embryonic body cavity lined with mesoderm.
coilos	G	Hollow, empty. MENINGOCOEL – a hernia of the meninges. See also **cele** and **kele**.
coinos	G	Common. COENOBIUM – a group of independent cells living within a common envelope.
col		See **con, colon**.
coleon	G	A sheath, scabbard. COLEOCYSTITIS – inflammation of the vagina and bladder.
colicos	G	Having pain in the colon; colic. COLIC.
colla	G	Glue. COLLOID.
collum	L	The neck. TORTICOLLIS – wry, twisted neck.
collutum	L	Washed, rinsed. COLLUTORY – of a mouth-wash or gargle. See also **luo**.
colobo	G	Truncated, curtailed, mutilated. COLOBOMA – defect of one of the tissues of the eye, e.g., the iris.
colon	G	The colon. COLON.
colostra, colostrum	L	The first milk after a birth. COLOSTRUM.

colpos	G	The bosom, vagina, womb; fistulous ulcer. COLPORRHAPHY – vaginal suture.
com		See **con**.
comedo, comidones	L	A glutton, gluttons. COMEDO – a blackhead.
comizo	G	To take care of. NOSOCOMIAL – of a disease originating or arising in a hospital.
con	L	Together with, in combination. CONJUGAL – pertaining to marriage and to the husband and wife pair.
conche	G	A mussel, cockle, shaped so. CONCHAE – various anatomical structures shaped like a shell, e.g., in the nose.
concipio, conceptum	L	To contain, take in, become pregnant, experience. CONCEPTION – fertilization of the ovum leading to pregnancy. Also, an idea.
condylos	G	The knob of a joint, knuckle. CONDYLE.
conis	G	Dust. PNEUMOCONIOSIS – affection of the lung usually by coal or stone dusts.
cono	G	Pine cone, a cone. LENTICONUS – a conical projection of the eye lens.
contra	L	Against, opposite. CONTRALATERAL – on the other side of the body. Cf. ipsilateral.
copos	G	Toil, pain, fatigue, weariness. COPIOPIA – eye fatigue.
copros	G	Dung, faeces. COPROPORPHYRIN – porphyrin in the faeces.
copto	G	To strike, knock, smite. SYNCOPE – fainting or sudden loss of consciousness or strength.
cor, cordis	L	1. The heart. CORDATE – heart shaped. 2. See **chorde**.
coracoeides	G	Shaped like a crow's beak. CORACOID. See also **corone**.
core	G	A maiden, puppet, the eye pupil. ANISOCORIA – having unequal eye pupils.
corium	L	Hide, leather. EXCORIATION – removal of the epidermmis or skin.
cormos	G	The trunk of a lopped tree. CAMPTOCORMIA – a

deformity in which the body inclines forwards.

corneus	L	Horny, or horn-like substance. CORNEA – the outer transparent covering of the eye.
cornu	L	Horn shaped. BICORNUATE – having two horn-shaped parts.
corona	L	A crown, a garland, an encircling structure; the crown of the head. CORONAL – pertaining to the crown of the head and especially the planes parallel to the coronal suture and at right angles to the sagittal plane.
corone	G	A crow, shaped like a crow's beak. CORONOID – the mandibular process. See also **coracoeides**.
coros	G	Satiety, surfeit. ACORIA – not feeling satiated after feeding.
corpus	L	A body; substance. CORPORAL, CORPOREAL.
cortex, corticis	L	Bark, rind. CORTICAL – applied to the outer layer of an organ, e.g., the cerebrum.
coryne	G	Club, shepherd's staff, knobbly shoots on a plant. CORYNEBACTERIA – a group of bacteria, some of which are club-chaped.
coryza	G	Mucus from the nose. CORYZA – the common cold.
costa	L	A rib. COSTAL.
cotyle	G	Cup-shaped, hollow, a socket. COTYLOID – a cup-like hollow, e.g., that of the acetabulum, q.v.
coxa	L	The hip-bone. MEROCOXALGIA – pain in the thigh and hip.
cranion	G	The skull. CRANIUM.
crasis	G	A mixing, combination, a proper mixture. DYSCRASIA – illness, a pathological condition.
cratos	G	Power, strength, might. ACRATIA – loss of strength.
creas	G	Flesh, meat, carcass. CREATINE – a compound found in muscles.
cremaster	G	A suspender; the muscles which suspend the testes. CREMASTER.
crena	L?	A notch, cog, space between two holes in a strap. CRENATED – having a notched or scalloped edge or surface.

crene	G	A well, spring. CRENOTHERAPY – treatment by the waters at Spas.
cresco; **crescentia**	L	To come into existence, grow; an increase. EXCRESCENCE – an outgrowth, normal or abnormal.
cribrum	L	A sieve. CRIBRIFORM – with many perforations.
cricos	G	A ring. CRICOID – annular.
crino	G	To pick out, to separate. EXOCRINE – applied to a gland secreting into a duct.
crisis	G	A separation, judgement, trial, dispute. PARAECCRISIS – disturbed secretion or excretion.
crista	L	The crest of a bird or of a helmet. CRISTA – a crest or ridge usually on a bone.
crotaphos	G	A clapping, rattling noise. DICROTIC – applied to a pulse wave with a double peak.
crotesis	G	Knocking. GONYCROTESIS – knock-kneed (*genu valgum*).
crus	L	The shin, tibia. CRUS.
cryos	G	Frost, icy cold. CRYOGENIC – producing low temperature.
cryptos	G	Hidden, latent, secret. CRYPTORCHIDISM – undescended testis.
cum		See **con**.
cuneus	L	A wedge, shaped so. CUNEIFORM – wedge-shaped.
curro; cursum	L	To run, move quickly; moved. PRECURSOR – something occurring first.
cuspis	L	A point, especially of a spear. BICUSPID – with two projections.
cutis	L	The skin. CUTICULAR – pertaining to the skin.
cyanos	G	Dark blue enamel, lapsis lazuli, blue colour. CYANOSIS – the blueness associated with reduced haemoglobin.
cyclos	G	A circle, cycle; around. CYCLOTHYMIA – having alternating periods of depression and elation.
cyeo, cyo	G	To conceive, be impregnated. CYOGENIC – causing pregnancy.
cyesis	G	Pregnancy. ACYESIS – female sterility, non-pregnancy.

cyllos	G	Crooked, crippled, club-footed. CYLLOSIS – club-foot.
cyon, cyno	G	A dog or bitch, a hound, watch-dog. CYNOCEPHALIC – with a head shaped like a dog's.
cyrtos, cyrtosis	G	Convex, bulging, hump-backed in the cervical region. See **kyphos.**
cystis	G	The bladder. CYSTITIS – inflammation of the bladder.
cytos	G	A hollow vessel or structure. CYTOLOGY – the study of cells.

D

dacryon	G	A tear, drop. DACRYOCYSTITIS – inflammation of the lacrimal sac.
dactylos	G	A digit; the breadth of a finger. POLYDACTYLY – having an excess number of digits.
dartos	G	Flayed; skin flayed from an animal. DARTOS – the contractile tunica around the testes.
de	L	1. Away from. DECIDUA – the membrance lost from the uterus after parturition. 2. See **deo**
decusso	L	To divide diagonally to form the letter X. DECUSSATE – to cross over forming an X-shape. Cf. **chiasma.**
defero	L	To carry away, transport. DUCTUS DEFERENS – the vas deferens. (See **de** and **fero**)
deire, dere	G	The neck or throat. DERENCEPHALOCOEL – a protrusion of brain tissue through one or more of the cervical vertebrae.
delos	G	Conspicuous, clear, manifest. ADELOMORPHIC – amorphous.
delphys	G	The uterus. SYNADELPHUS – a foetal monster with two fused bodies. See **adelphos**
delta; deltoides	G	The Greek letter delta; shaped so. DELTOID – triangular in shape.
demos	G	A district, people inhabiting a district. EPIDEMIC –

a disease with temporarily high incidence.

dendreon, **dendron**	G	A tree, shaped so. DENDRITE – one of the afferent branching processes of a nerve cell.
dens; dentis	L	A tooth; of it. DENTINE – the hard material of teeth.
deo	G	To bind, tie, fetter. ARTHRODESIS – deliberate ankylosis of a joint. See **desmos.**
deon	G	That which is proper, needful, right. DEONTOLOGY – the study of professional duties and ethics.
der		See **deire.**
derma	G	Skin, hide. DERMATOPHYTE – a skin fungus.
desis		See **deo.**
desmos	G	A binding, fetter, latch. DESMOSOME – an organelle thought to link cells together. See **deo.**
deuteros	G	Second, next. DEUTERANOPIA – loss of vision of two of the primary colours.
dexis	G	A bite, biting. LYSSODEXIS – a rabid bite.
dexter	L	On the righthand side. DEXTROCARDIA – with the heart displaced towards the right.
di(a)	G	1. Through, over. DIARRHOEA – abnormally frequent passage of liquid faeces from the gut. 2. See **dis.**
diairesis	G	Divisibility, dissection, distribution. DIAERESIS – the separation of two parts normally united. Cf. **airesis.**
dian		See **dies.**
diapeiresis		See **peiro.**
diaphoresis	G	Evaporation, perspiration. DIAPHORESIS – profuse sweating.
diastema	G	An interval, distance, aperture. DIASTEMA – the space between two structures, e.g., adjacent teeth.
diastole	G	A dilation. DIASTOLE – dilation of the heart on refilling.
dicha, dichos	G	Sundered in two, doubly, in two ways. DICHOTOMY – division into two.
diclis	G	Double fold, folding doors. TYPHLODICLIDITIS – inflammation of the ileocaecal valve.

didymoi	G	1. Twins. ISCHIODIDYMIC – applied to twins fused at the pelvis. 2. Testes, ovaries. EPIDIDYMIS – the tubular organ above, beside and below the testis.
dies	L	Daytime, the day. CIRCADIAN – pertaining to the 24 hour period of a day and a night. See **diurnus** and **nox.**
digitus	L	A finger or toe. DIGITIFORM – having the shape of fingers.
dine	G	A rotation, whirling. OTICODINIA – vertigo, dizziness from ear disease.
dioptricos	G	The science of DIOPTRICS, i.e., the use of lenses.
diploos	G	Double, two fold. DIPLOCOCCUS – bacteria often appearing double by not fully separating after subdivision.
dipsa	G	Thirst. DIPSOMANIA – excessive desire to drink; also alcoholism.
dis	G	Twice, doubly. DIPLEGIA – bilateral paralysis.
discos	G	A quoit or disc; shaped so. DISCOPLACENTA – a disc-shaped placenta.
diurnus	L	Lasting for a day, daily. DIURNAL – pertaining to events occurring during the day (and not the night). See **dies** and **nox.**
dochos	G	Containing, holding. CHOLEDOCHOLITHIASIS – stone in the bile duct.
docimasia	G	Examination, test. DOCIMASIA.
dolor	L	Pain, ache, grief. DOLOR, DOLOUR.
dontos		See **odont.**
dorsum	L	The back. DORSAL – pertaining to the back.
dosis	G	A gift, contribution, dose. ANTIDOTE – combating the effect of a dose of poison or disease.
drepane	G	A sickle or pruning-hook; shaped so. DREPANOCYTE – a sickle-shaped red cell in the blood.
dromos	G	A race, run. PRODROMAL – precursal, premonitory.
duco; ductum	L	To lead; led. DUCT.
duo	L	Two. DUOPARENTAL – pertaining to derivation from two sexes or two parents.

duodecim	L	Twelve. DUODENUM – the part of the gut distal to the stomach, about twelve inches long.
durus	L	Tough, hard. DURA mater – the outer meninx covering the brain.
dys	G	Bad, unfortunate. DYSPEPSIA – poor digestion, indigestion after eating.

E

e		See **ex** L.
eburneus	L	Made of ivory. EBURNATION – bone or dentine exposed, transformed and polished.
ec	G	From, out of. CIRSECTOMY – removal of part of varicose veins. See **ectome**.
echinos	G	Sea-urchin, hedgehog. ECHINOCYTE – a cell with many points, a burr cell.
echo	G	To hold, have. MEIONECTIC – blood less saturated than normal at a given tension of oxygen.
eclampsis	G	Sudden development, shining forth. ECLAMPSIS – a sudden convulsion, with or without coma.
eco		See **oicos**.
ectasis	G	An extension, stretching. LYMPHANGIECTASIS – dilation of the lymphatic vessels.
ectic		See **echo**.
ectome	G	An excision, removal, castration. MASTECTOMY – removal of a breast.
ectos	G	Outside, outwith. ECTODERM – the outer cell layer of the embryo.
ectroma	G	An untimely birth. Now: abnormality or congenital absence of something in a foetus. ECTROMELIA – absence of one or more limb bones.
ectropion	G	Eversion of the eyelid. ECTROPION.
ectrosis	G	Miscarriage. ECTROSIS – abortion; also treatment which arrests the course of a disease.
eczema	G	A disease of the skin. ECZEMA.
edema		See **oidema**.
edentulus	L	Toothless. EDENTULOUS.

ef		See **ex** L.
effero	L	To carry outside, emit, carry away. EFFERENT – centrifugal, opposite to afferent.
ego	G,L	I, myself. EGOCENTRIC – self-centred.
eicon	G	An image, semblance. ISEICONIA, ISOICONIA – having equal images in both eyes.
eidetic	G	Constituting an image. See **eidos**.
eidolon	G	A likeness, mental image. See **idea** and **eidos**.
eidos	G	A form, particular kind, type. ODONTOID – tooth-like.
eileos, ileos	G	1. Intestinal obstruction. ILEUS – colic. 2. See **ile, ilia**.
elaion	G	Olive oil, butter, fat. Now associated with fat in obesity. ELAIOPATHY – a fatty oedema, especially in the leg joints.
elasma	G	Metal beaten flat; medical probes. XANTHELASMA – soft yellow plaques, especially on the eyelids.
elcos		See **helcos**.
electron	G	Amber (a substance used to demonstrate static electricity). ELECTROENCEPHALOGRAM – a recording of the electrical activity of the brain.
eleo		See **elaion**.
elytron	G	A sheath, a covering. CYSTOELYTROPLASTY – repair of damage to the bladder and vagina.
em		See **en**.
embolos	G	Something pointed which penetrates easily, a wedge, peg, or spear. EMBOLISM – a clot or plug sudddenly blocking a blood vessel.
embryon	G	One of the young; the foetus. EMBRYO. See also **em** and **bryo**.
emesis	G	Vomiting. EMETIC – a substance causing vomiting.
emmetria	G	Having a fit measure, i.e., in proper proportion. EMMETROPIA – optimum visual acuity.
emollio	L	To soften, make pliable, gentle, feminine. EMOLLIENT – a soothing, protective balm.
empyema	G	Abscess. EMPYEMA – an accumulation of pus in a body cavity, especially in the thorax

en	G	In, on. ENTHLASIS – skull fracture with depressed bone.
enantios	G	Opposite, opposed. ENANTIOPATHIA – a situation in which one disease cures another; such disease pairs.
encephalos	G	The brain, (within the head). ENCEPHALITIS – inflammation of the brain. See **cephale**.
enchyma	G	The filling or content of a vessel. Now, generalized tissue. PARENCHYMA – the specially functional tissue of an organ, not the **stroma**, q.v.
endon	G	Within, in the house or family. ENDODERM – the inner cell layer of the embryo.
endysis	G	Entry. CHOLECYSTENDYSIS – to probe into the gall bladder.
enieme	G	To send in, plunge in, implant. ENEMA – the injection of liquid into the rectum and distal colon; also the liquid injected.
ensis	L	A sword. ENSIFORM – sword-shaped. Cf. **xiphos**.
enteron	G	A piece of gut, the bowels. ENTERITIS – inflammation of the gut.
enthesis	G	An insertion, something put into the mouth. ENTHESIS – similar to prothesis, something artificial employed internally.
entos	G	Within, inside. ENTOCOEL – an internal hernia. See also **endon** and **intus**.
eo, itum	L	To go, went. INTROITUS – the entrance to the vaginia.
eos	G	The morning, daybreak, and thus the red colour of dawn. EOSIN – a red stain, used in histology.
ep		See **epi**.
ependyma	G	An upper garment. EPENDYMA – the epithelial lining of the cavities of the central nervous system.
ephelis	G	A freckle, rough spot on the face. EPHELIDES – freckles.
ep(i)	G	1. On, outside. EPIDERMIS – the outer layer of the skin. 2. Amongst. EPIDEMIC – a disease of temporarily high incidence.

epiphora	G	Persistent tears, floods of tears. EPIPHORA.
epiploon	G	A fold of the peritoneum, the omentum. EPIPLOON.
epision	G	The pubic region. EPISIOTOMY – incision of the vulva and/or perineum.
epithymia	G	Desire, lust: supposed to come from the solar plexus, and hence now used to mean this. ABEPITHYMIA – paralysis of the solar plexus.
erastes	G	One who loves, a lover of persons. PAEDERASTY – anal homosexual intercourse with a boy.
eremos	G	Lack or absence of something, a desert, solitude. CHOROIDEREMIA – degeneration of the choroid layer of the eye.
ereptomai	G	To feed on something. EREPSIN – a group of proteolytic enzymes in the small intestine.
eresis		See airesis and diairesis.
erethizo	G	To irritate, arouse, provoke. DYSERETHESIA – lack of sensitivity to stimuli.
ergon	G	Work, activity. CHOLINERGIC – applied to synapses utilizing acetyl choline as transmitter substance.
eructo	L	To belch forth, emit. ERUCTATION – belching.
eryo	G	To drag, tear away violently. PHACOERYSIS – removal of the eye lens.
erythema	G	Redness of the skin, flush. ERYTHEMA.
erythros	G	Red. ERYTHROCYTE – a red blood cell.
eschara	G	A fire-place, altar, burning coals in a brazier. Also the crust which forms on a cauterized wound. ESCHAR – a sloughing scar, usually after a burn, thermal or caustic.
esis		See hieme.
eso, eiso	G	Into, inside. ESOGASTRITIS – inflammation of the gastric mucosa.
esophagus		See oesophagus.
esthesia		See aisthesis.
ethmos	G	A strainer, sieve. ETHMOID – a bone with many perforations. Cf. cribriform.
ethnos	G	A company of people, a nation. ETHNOLOGY – the study of the races of mankind.

etio		See **aitia**.
eu	G	Well, normal. EUTHYROID – having normal thyroid function.
eune	G	The marriage bed. DYSPAREUNIA – difficult, painful coitus.
euphoria	G	Great wellbeing, cheerfulness. EUPHORIA.
euryno	G	To widen, dilate, clear a place. HYSTEREURYNTER – an instrument for widening the uterus opening.
eurys	G	Broad, wide. ANEURYSM – a dilation of a part of the circulatory system. See **euryno**.
ex	L	Out of. EXCISION – a cutting out.
exia, exis		See **hexis**.
ex(o)	G	1. See **ec**. 2. Outside. EXOPATHIC – of a disease originating outside the body.
extra	L	Outside. EXTRARENAL – not involving the kidney.

F

faba	L	The bean *Vicia fava*. FAVISM – haemolysis after ingestion of beans of this species.
facies	L	Form, appearance, face. CRANIOFACIAL – involving the face and skull.
facio; factum	L	To make, form; produced. ABORTIFACIENT – a substance used to provoke an abortion.
faction		See **facio**.
faex; faecis	L	Dregs, remains, refuse; of these. FAECES – undigested food remains.
falx, falcis	L	A sickle, shaped so. FALCIFORM – sickle-shaped.
farcio	L	To fill full, to cram. INFARCT – damage from ischaemia after obstruction of part of the circulation.
fascia	L	A band, bandage. FASCIORRHAPHY – repair of damaged fascia.
fascis; fasciculus	L	A bundle, packet; a little bundle or packet. FASCICULUS – a small group of nerve fibres or muscle fibres.

faux, fauces	L	The throat, gullet, narrow passages. FAUCES – the narrow part between the mouth and the pharynx.
favism		See **faba**.
favus	L	Hexagonal, like a honeycomb. FAVUS – a skin disease in which there are finally hexagonal crusts or plaques.
faveolus		A late form from **favus**.
febris	L	Fever. FEBRILE – feverish.
fenestra	L	Window, loop-hole. FENESTRATION – making an opening, or perforation.
fero	L	To bear, carry. SEMINIFEROUS – conveying or producing semen. See also **phero** and **phoreo**.
fetus	L	The bearing of young; the offspring. FETUS – in humans, the young *in utero*, after 7 or 8 weeks of development.
fibra	L	A fibre. FIBROUS.
fibrilla	L	A small fibre. FIBRIL.
fibula	L	A pin, bolt, brooch. FIBULA – the minor bone of the crus. Cf. **perone**.
fic		See **facio**.
fid		See **findo**.
filum	L	A thread or cord. FILIFORM – threadlike.
fimbriae	L	The fringe, loose border or edge of something. FIMBRIAE – fringes on a rim or a surface.
findo; fidi	L	To split; split. BIFID – split in two, V-shaped. Cf. **furcate**.
fissum		See **findo**.
fistula	L	A tube, pipe. FISTULA – an abnormal opening, often experimental
flaccidus	L	Withered, flabby, languid. FLACCID – relaxed, soft, weak.
flatus	L	A blowing, blast. FLATUS – gas from the gut or the lungs.
flavus	L	Yellow. FLAVOPROTEIN – a compound containing the yellow substance flavin.
flecto; flexum	L	To bend, curl, curve; bent, curved. FLEXION – bending, bent.

fluo; fluxum	L	To flow, run, stream, exude; flowed. FLUID.
folium	L	A leaf. EXFOLIATION – a special form of desquamation at birth; a sloughing of surface cells.
foramen	L	An opening, hole. FORAMEN MAGNUM – the large opening at the base of the skull.
foris	L	An opening, door. PERFORATION.
forma	L	Shape, likeness, form. FILIFORM – thread-like.
fornix	L	An arch, a vault. FORNIX – part of the fore-brain, of an arched shape.
fosssa	L	A ditch, channel. FOSSA – a hollow.
fovea	L	A pit. FOVEA – applied to various small pits or depressions in the body, especially that of the retina.
foveola	L	A small pit. FOVEOLAE GASTRICAE – small pits in the gastric mucosa, the gastric pits.
fract		See **frango**.
frango; fractum	L	To break; smashed. FRACTURE.
fremitus	L	A low murmur, growling noise. FREMITUS – a vibration, usually in the chest.
frenum	L	A bridle, mechanism of restraint. FRENULUM – a small fold of skin or mucous membrane which limits movement.
frons; frontis	L	The forehead, brow. FRONTAL.
fuga; fugax	L	Flight, fleeting. FUGUE – a transient period of immediate amnesia. See **fugio**.
fugio	L	To flee. CENTRIFUGAL – moving away from the centre. Cf. **phyge**.
fulgur	L	A flash of lightning. FULGURANT – electic spark discharges used to make lesions.
fulmino	L	To strike with lightning. FULMINANT – progressing very quickly to a crisis. See **fulgur**.
funct		See **fungor**.
fundo; fusum	L	To pour; poured out. INFUSION – an aqueous extract which can be given intravenously by gravity.
fundus	L	The base or bottom of something. FUNDUS.
fungor; functus	L	To be busy, to perform; done. MALFUNCTION – working improperly.
funis; funiculus	L	A rope, cord; a thin string. FUNICULITIS – inflam-

mation of a cord-like structure, e.g., the spermatic cord or spinal nerves.

furca   L   A two-pronged fork. BIFURCATE – with two branches, Y-shaped. Cf. **findo.**

furfur   L   Bran, scurf on the skin. DEFURFURATION – loss of epidermal cells as dandruff.

furunculus   L   A protruberance left after pruning, a knob. FURUNCLE – a boil.

fus   See **fundo** or **fusus.**

fuscus   L   Dark in colour, blank. LINEA FUSCA – a dark line from navel to pubis.

fusus   L   A spindle; a cylinder of bars used for winding rope on. FUSIFORM – spindle-shaped.

G

gala; galactos   G   Milk; milky. GALATOSE – milk sugar.

galea   L   A helmet, shaped so. GALEATUS – born with a caul.

gamos   G   Marriage, a wedding. GAMETE – a haploid reproductive cell.

ganglion   G   An encysted swelling on a tendon. Now, a knot of tissue, usually nervous. GANGLION.

gangraina   G   Gangrene. GANGRENE.

gaster, gastros   G   The paunch, belly, shaped so. Now the stomach. GASTRITIS – inflammation of the stomach.

gelo   L   1. To freeze. GELOSIS – a hard lump, often in a muscle.
2. See **gelos.**

gelos   G   Laughter. GELOTHERAPY – treatment by causing laughter.

geminus   L   A twin. GEMINI – twins.

gemma   L   A bud. PERIGEMMAL – surrounding a taste-bud.

gen   See **genesis, genos, genus** or **gonos.**

gena   L   The cheek, side of the face. GENAL – pertaining to the cheek. Cf. **genys.**

geneion   G   The part of the face covered by the beard, the chin. GENIOPLASTY – plastic surgery of the chin.

genesis	G	Origin, beginning, producing, creating. NEOGENESIS – creation of something new.
genit		See **gigno.**
genos	G	Race, offspring, generation. GENOCIDE – the destruction of a race of mankind.
genu	L	The knee, bent as a knee. GENU.
genus; generis	L	Race, kind; of these. GENUS – a taxonomic group between the family and the species.
genys	G	The side of the face, the cheek, the jaw. GENYANTRALGIA – pain in the maxillary sinus.
geras	G	Old age. GERIATRICS – medical care of old people.
germen; germinis	L	An embryo, a sprout, bud; of these. GERMINAL – associated with a source of new cells or tissue.
gero; gestum	L	To carry around, bear a child; that which is borne. GESTATION – the period of pregnancy.
geron	G	Old man, elder. GERONTOLOGY – the study of old age.
gesto, gestum		See **gero.**
geuma; geusis	G	Taste; the sense of taste. ALLOTRIOGEUSTIA – an abnormal sense of taste.
gibbus	L	Humped. GIBBOUS – convex, protuberant.
gigno; genitum	L	To bear, conceive; begotten. GENITAL – pertaining to the sex-organs.
gingiva	L	The gums (of the teeth). GINGIVITIS – inflammation of these.
ginglymos	G	A hinge. GINGLYMUS – a hinge joint, e.g., the elbow.
glandulae	L	Originally small acorn-shaped objects, and thus used of the glands of the neck and throat, especially when swollen. Hence similar structures. GLANDULAR.
glans	L	An acorn, shaped so. GLANS PENIS.
glaucos	G	Gleaming, with a clear sheen; a bluish-green colour. GLAUCOMA – eye diseases which often lead to a characteristic sheen in the eye, variously described as grey, bluish or greenish.
glene	G	The eyeball; or a shallow socket. GLENOID – socket-like.

gleucos	G	Sweet new wine, sweetness. GLUCOSE – a sugar. Cf. **glycys**.
glia; gloios	G	Glue; glutinous. GLIOMA – a tumour of glial tissue.
glomus	L	A skein of yarn. GLOMERULUS – a tangle of blood vessels; e.g., that adjacent to Bowman's capsule in the kidney.
glossa	G	The tongue. GLOSSOPHARYNGEAL – appertaining to the tongue and pharynx.
glottis	G	The opening into the trachea. GLOTTIS.
gloutos	G	A buttock, rump. GLUTEAL – pertaining to the buttocks.
gluco		See **gleucos** or **glycys**.
glutino	L	To glue together. AGGLUTINATION – small particles sticking together to make relatively large masses.
glutio	L	To swallow. DEGLUTITION – swallowing.
glycys	G	Sweet. GLYCOGEN – the carbohydrate, consisting of polymerized glucose, stored in many animals. Cf. **gleucos**.
glypho	G	To carve, engrave, incise. DERMATOGLYPHICS – the science of the skin ridges, especially those on hands and feet.
gnathos	G	The jaw. GNATHOPLASTY – plastic repair of the jaw and cheek.
gnome	G	Thought, judgement, intention. See **gnomon** and **gnosis**.
gnomon	G	One who discerns, an expert, a witness, a mark. PATHOGNOMONIC – applied to a diagnostic sign or symptom of a disease.
gnosis	G	A search for knowledge. DIAGNOSIS – elucidation of the nature of a disease.
gnotos	G	Understood, known. GNOTOBIOTIC – describing experimental animals harbouring only known microorganisms.
gomphosis	G	A bolting together to form a framework. GOMPHOSIS – a peg-and-socket joint secured by fibrous tissue, especially those of the teeth.
gonad		See **gone**.

gone	G	Offspring, race, family, seed. GONECYSTITIS – inflammation of the seminal vesicle. See **genos, gonos.**
gonia	G	An angle or corner; a joint. GONIOSCOPE – an instrument for examining the angle of the anterior eye chamber. Cf. **genu.**
gonos	G	Child, offspring, race, begetting, genitals. GONORRHOEA – a venereal disease. See **genos, gone.**
gony	G	The knee. GONARTHROSIS – arthritic disease of the knee. Cf. **genu , gonia.**
gradior	L	To walk, step, stride. ANTEGRADE, ANTEROGRADE – progressing in the normal direction; opposite to retrograde.
gramma	G	Something written or drawn. CARDIOGRAM – a record of the activity of the heart.
granum	L	A grain, a small particle. GRANULOCYTE – a cell with grains in its cytoplasm; usually refers to a leucocyte.
graphe	G	A drawing or inscription. CARDIOGRAPH – an instrument to record the activity of the heart.
gravis	L	Heavy. See **gravidus.**
gravidus	L	Pregnant. MULTIGRAVIDA – a woman who has been pregnant more than once.
griseus	L	Grey, bluish-grey. SUBSTANTIA GRISEA – grey matter of the central nervous system.
grumus	L	A little heap, a hillock. GRUMOUS, GRUMOSE – clotted, lumpy.
grypos; gryposis	G	Aquiline, hooked; hooking of the nails. ONYCHOGRYPOSIS – curved, or ingrown nails.
gubernaculum	L	A rudder; direction, management. GUBERNACULUM – that which guides; usually applied to the ligaments controlling the descent of the testes into the scrotum.
gustatus	L	Taste, the sense of taste. GUSTATORY – applied to the sense of taste. Cf. **geuma.**
guttur	L	Throat, windpipe. GUTTUROTETANY – a guttural spasm.

gyne; gynaicos G A woman, wife; feminine. GYNAECOLOGY – the study of diseases of the female genital tract.

gyros G A ring, round in shape. GYRECTOMY – excision of part of a cerebral gyrus.

H

habena; habenula L A thong or rein to hold something. HABENULAE – small retaining structures; also various small projections and other structures.

haemato See **haima**.

haima; haimatos G Blood; bloody. HAEMATOLOGY – the study of blood.

halismos G Sprinkled with salt. See **hals**.

halitus L Breath, vapour. HALITOSIS – malodorous breath.

halo L 1. To breathe, emit vapour, be fragrant. INHALATION – a breath taken in.
2. See **hals** or **halos**.

halos G A circular area or object, a halo, the ciliary body of the eye. HALO – circular imprint of the ciliary processes on the vitreous humour. Also a coloured ring seen in glaucoma, or that round the macula lutea.

hals G A lump of salt. HALISTERESIS – loss of calcareous salts from bones, osteomalacia.

hama G At once, simultaneously. HAMARTHRITIS – generalized arthritis.

hamartano G To fail, err, do wrong. HAMARTOMA – a benign hypertrophy of normal tissue forming a nodule.

hamus, hamulus L A hook, a fish hook, a little hook. HAMATE – hook-shaped.

haphe G The sense of touch, contact, grip. PARAPHIA – a disturbed sense of touch. See also **hapto**.

haploos G Single, simple. HAPLOID – a cell with only one genome.

hapsis G Touching, contact. See **hapto**.

hapto G To join, grasp, fasten, touch. HAPTOMETER – an instrument to measure touch sensitivity. See also **haphe**.

haustrum	L	An irrigation device, with small buckets. HAUSTRA – sacculations or recesses, especially in the colon.
hebe	G	Youth, young man; the time of puberty, pubes. HEBEPHRENIA – a type of schizophrenia with childish behaviour.
hedone	G	Delight, pleasure. HYPHEDONIA – reduced appreciation of pleasurable sensations. (Better: hypohedonia.)
helcos	G	A wound, ulcer. HELCOSIS – ulceration.
helios	G	The sun. HELIOSIS – sunstroke.
helix; helicos	G	A twist, whorl, convolution; coiled. HELICAL.
helmins	G	An intestinal worm, flat or round. HELMINTHIASIS – infected with worms.
helos	G	A nail-head, stud, wart, callus. HELOTOMY – cutting or removal of corns or callouses.
hem		See haima.
hemera	G	Day, daylight. HEMERALOPIA – poor sight or blindness in daylight. This word is sometimes wrongly used to mean its opposite, night blindness, nyctalopia. This is a mistake because the root words are hemera, alaos, opia: day-time, blind, seeing. See alaos.
hemi	G	A combining prefix indicating half. HEMIPARESIS – muscular weakness on one side of the body.
hepar; hepatos	G	The liver; pertaining to it. HEPATIC.
heres; hereditas	L	An heir; an inheritance. HEREDITY.
hermeneia	G	Interpretation, explanation, expression. HERMENEUTIC – pertaining to interpretation.
herpes; herpetos	G	Shingles; of it. See herpo.
herpo	G	To creep, move slowly. HERPANGINA – a virus infection of the throat and/or soft palate, with sudden onset and short duration.
heteros	G	The other one, not the usual one. HETERODONT – having different types of teeth.
hexis	G	Possessing a state or condition of the body or

mind. PLEIONEXIA – a condition in which the blood is more saturated than normal at a given oxygen tension.

hiatus	L	An opening, gap, cleft. HIATUS.
hidros	G	Sweat, exudation. BROMHIDROSIS – stinking sweat. Sometimes wrongly: bromidrosis.
hiemi, hienai	G	To let go, release. PARESIS – some degree of paralysis or muscular weakness.
hieron		See hieros.
hieros	G	Divine, holy, sacred. PLATYHIERIC – with a wide sacrum. Cf sacer.
hilum	L	A little thing, trifle. HILUM – a depression where vessels enter an organ.
hippocampus	G	A mythical sea-monster like a horse with a fish's tail. HIPPOCAMPUS – a part of the forebrain thought to resemble the monster in shape.
hircus	L	A male goat; its smell. HIRCISMUS – the odour from decomposing sweat in the axilla.
histo		See histos.
histos	G	A loom, weaving, web. HISTOLYSIS – the breakdown of tissue.
histrio	L	An actor, boaster. HISTRIONIC – having exaggerated gestures or mannerisms.
hizano	G	To settle down, sit. Now, to sit fast. MYOSYNIZESIS – muscular adhesions.
hodos	G	The way, manner of doing things, path. HODONEUROMERE – a segment of the embryonic nervous system with its paired spinal nerves.
holos	G	Whole, entire, complete. HOLOCRINE – a gland which sheds the cells containing the secretion of the gland.
homales	G	Level, even. HOMALOCEPHALUS – having a flattened head.
homeo		See homoios.
homo; hominis	L	A human being; human. HOMINID – belonging to the family Hominidae.
homoios	G	Alike, equal. HOMOIOTHERM – an animal with a nearly constant body temperature, opposite to

poikilotherm. Sometimes improperly spelt homotherm. See **homos**.

homologos G Agreeing with, corresponding. HOMOLOGY – morphological and evolutionary correspondence.

homos G Common to, the same. HOMOGENETIC – having a common descent or origin.

hordeum L Barley (seed). HORDEOLUM – a stye on the eyelid.

hormao G To start, begin something. HORMION – the medial anterior point of the spheno-occipital bone.

horme G An impulse, assault, onrush, a strong attack. HORMONE – a product of endocrine glands, and similar activating metabolites.

humerus L Originally "umerus". The shoulder. Later, the upper part of the arm. HUMERUS. See **omos, 1**.

humor L Originally "umor". Wetness, humidity, moisture. Later: one of the four basic moods or temperaments. HUMORAL – applied to fluid or gel secretions; e.g., the aqueous humour.

hy G Shaped like the Greek letter upsilon, Y. HYOID – a bone at the base of the tongue shaped like this.

hyalos G Crystalline stone, glass. HYALINE – clear, transparent.

hydatis G Watery vesicle. HYDATIFORM – vesicular in shape. See also **hydor**.

hydor G Water, watery. HYDRAGOGUE – producing a watery discharge.

hydrargyros G 'Liquid silver', mercury. HYDRARGYRIA – mercury poisoning.

hydrops G Dropsy. HYDROPOTHERAPY – treatment with ascitic fluid.

hygieia G Healthy in body or mind. HYGIENE.

hygros G Liquid, moist, over-flowing. HYGROBLEPHARIC – pertaining to the ducts of the lacrimal glands.

hyle G,L Trees, wood, material, matter. HYLOTROPY – phase changes in matter.

hymen G Thin skin, a membrane, parchment. HYMENOTOMY – the cutting of the hymen.

hyper	G	Above, beyond. HYPERCAPNIA – with excess carbon dioxide in the blood
hyphaimos	G	Blood-shot, suffused with blood. HYPHAEMA – bleeding in the anterior chamber of the eye.
hyphe	G	A web, something woven. HYPHEPHILIA – sexual pleasure from fabrics.
hypnos	G	Sleep. HYPNOSIS – an induced lack of consciousness resembling a sleeping state.
hyp(o)	G	Under, below. HYPOXIA – with less than normal oxygen in the blood.
hypsi		See **hypsos**.
hypsos	G	Height, the summit, the crown. HYPSONOSUS – mountain sickness.
hystera	G	The uterus. HYSTERECTOMY – removal of the uterus.

I

iamatos	G	Of remedies, medicines. IAMATOLOGY – the study of remedies.
iaomai	G	To heal, cure. See **iasis**.
iasis	G	From **iaomai**. Now used as the suffix of disease names. LITHIASIS – a disease in which concretions are deposited in various places in the body.
iathenai	G	To be cured, healed. IATHERGY – the immunity of a person desensitized to the tuberculin skin test.
iatricos	G	Skilled in medical arts. See **iatros**.
iatros	G	A physician, healer. IATROGENIC – concerned with the (adverse) effects of a physician's efforts.
ichor	G	The watery liquid found in the blood vessels of the gods; thin watery serous fluid from sores. ICHORAEMIA – septicaemia.
ichthys	G	A fish. ICHTHYOSIS – dryness or scaliness of the skin.
icon		See **eicon**.
icteros	G	Jaundice, and the yellow colour associated with

		this disease. ICTERIC – pertaining to jaundice, affected by jaundice.
ictus	L	A blow, thrust, stab, stroke. ICTUS – a seizure or stroke.
idea	G	The form, ideal form, kind, sort. IDEOMOTOR – of the involuntary motor repsonse to an idea. See also **eidos**.
idios	G	Belonging to oneself, separate. IDIOPATHY – an illness arising "spontaneously", i.e., of unknown cause.
idros		See **hidros**.
il		See **in**.
ile, ilia	L	1. The loin, intestines. ILEOPROCTOSTOMY – an opening between ileum and rectum. 2. See also **eileos**.
ilis	L	A suffix indicating that which is done to something, the passive character of something. DUCTILIS – forming a duct.
im		See **in**.
impar	L	Unequal, uneven. IMPAR – unpaired, azygous.
in	L	1. Into, within. INHALATION – breathing in. 2. Not, negative. INVALID – not valid; not well or strong.
incos, incudo		See **incus**.
incus	L	An anvil. INCUS – bone of the middle ear, shaped like an anvil.
indusium	L	An outer tunic. INDUSIUM – an enclosing membrane, especially the amnion.
inferus	L	Below, lower. INFERIOR.
infra	L	Below, under. INFRASPINOUS – below the spine (of the scapula).
infundibulum	L	A funnel or hopper. INFUNDIBULUM – a funnel-shaped structure, especially the hypophyseal stalk.
inguen	L	The groin. INGUEN.
inion	G	The occipital bone, the occiput. INION – the occipital protuberance.
inos		See **is**.

insula	L	An island. INSULIN – one of the hormones secreted by the islets of Langerhans of the pancreas.
inter	L	Between, among. INTERARTICULAR – between articular surfaces.
intra	L	Inside. INTRACELLULAR – within a cell.
intus	L	Within, inside. INTUSSUSCEPTION – prolapse of one part of the intestine longitudinally into an adjacent part; also a process of protoplasmic growth by absorption of material at a molecular or microscopical level, not by apposition. Cf. **entos** and **endon**.
ipse	L	Self, oneself; used to give emphasis to the word it is prefixed to. IPSILATERAL – on the same side, opposite to contralateral.
ir		See **in** or **iris**.
iris, iridos	G	The rainbow, of similarly coloured things. IRIS – the coloured annular muscle around the pupil of the eye.
is; inos	G	Sinew, fibrous structures; of these. INOSAEMIA – excess of fibrinogen in the blood.
ischion	G	The hip-joint, the haunch. ISCHIORECTAL – concerned with the rectum and the ischial bone of the hip.
ischo	G	To restrain, hold, keep back. ISCHAEMIA – having an inadequate blood supply.
isis		See **osis**.
isos	G	Equal. ISOMORPHIC – of the same shape.
iter		See **eo**.
ithys	G	Straight. ITHYLORDOSIS – lordosis without any lateral bending.
itis	G	A suffix originally used to mean a disease, but later applied more specifically to inflammations. CYSTITIS – inflammation of the bladder.
itus		See **eo**.
ixos	G	Mistletoe, sticky bird-lime prepared from this, or like this. IXODES – a parasitic tick which attaches itself to humans.
izano, izesis	G	See **hizano**.

J

jacio; jactum	L	To throw; thrown. INJECTION.
jact		From **jacio**. JACTATION, JACTITATION – the restlessness of an acutely sick person.
jecur	L	The liver. JECUR.
jejunus	L	Fasting, hungry, meagre. Later empty. JEJUNUM – the gut between the duodenum and the ileum.
jugulum	L	The throat. JUGULAR – the main vein of the neck.
jugum	L	A yoke, usually joining two beasts. JUGUM – a ridge or groove connecting two structures or places.
jungo; junctum	L	To join two things together; joined. CONJUCTIVA – the membrane covering the opposed surfaces of the eye and eyelids.
jus	L	A broth, juice, soup. JUSCULUM – soup or broth.
juxta	L	Close to, near, hard by. JUXTAGLOMERULAR – adjacent to the glomerulus.

K

kali, kalium	A,L	Alkali. Now, potassium. HYPOKALAEMIA – abnormally low potassium concentration in the blood.
karyon	G	A nut, kernal. MEGAKARYOCYTE – a ceil with a large nucleus, found in bone marrrow.
keiro	G	To cut off one's hair, usually in mourning. KEIROSPASM – "barber's hand": involuntary spasms in the arm and hand muscles.
kele	G	A tumour, swelling. See also **cele**. KELOID – a kind of scar which enlarges and contains much collagen.
kenos	G	Empty, void. GASTRALGOKENOSIS – acute pain when the stomach is empty.
keras, keration	G	A horn, a little horn. Also, horny substance or horn-shaped. Now including the cornea of the eye. KERATOME – a knife for incising the cornea.
kern	D	A nucleus, kernal. KERNICTERUS – disease, espe-

cially of the new-born, in which the basal ganglia are yellow from bilirubin deposits.

keto D Associated with acetone (aketon, keton). KETOGENIC – forming ketone bodies in metabolism. Cf. **acetum.**

kineo G To move, set in motion. KINEMATICS – the science of motion.

kinesis G Movement, motion, change. KINESIOLOGY – the study of human movements.

kion G Uvula, especially when inflamed. KIOTOMY – cutting the uvula. Better: kionotomy. See **cion.**

klasis See **clasis.**

kleio G To shut, close. ARTHROKLEISIS – ankylosis of a joint. Cf. **ankylos.**

knephas G Twilight at dusk and dawn. AKNEPHASCOPIA – poor vision in dim light or twilight.

koilos G Hollow, concave. See also **coilos.** KOILONYCHIA – having concave nails, "spoon" nails.

kophos G Dull, dumb, deaf. LOGOKOPHOSIS – the condition of lacking comprehension of spoken language.

krauros G Brittle, friable. KRAUROSIS – the condition of being dry and shrivelled, especially of the vulva.

kyllos G Club-footed, deformed, crooked, crippled. KYLLOSIS – with a deformed foot, "club-foot".

kyma G A swelling, wave, swell. MYOKYMIA – persistent quivering of muscles.

kyphos G Bent forward, hunch-backed. KYPHOSIS – with abnormal posterior convexity of the thoracic spine, hunch-backed. See also **cyrtos.**

L

labium L A lip. LABIAL – pertaining to the lip.
labor L To glide, slip, fall down. LABILE – not fixed, sliding.
lac; lactis L Milk; milky. LACTATION – secretion of milk.
lacero L To tear to pieces. LACERATE.
lacerta L A lizard. Also used for the upper arm and its mus-

cles; later used for other groups of muscles, perhaps because of some fancied resemblance to a lizard or its muscles. LACERTUS – the fibrous attachment of some muscles.

lachrys		See **lacrima.**
lacrima	L	A tear (from the eye). LACRIMAL – appertaining to tears.
lacus	L	A lake, pool. LACUS – the inner corner of the eye.
lagos	G	A hare. LAGOPHTHALMOS – a condition in which complete closure of the eye is not possible.
laleo	G	To chatter, talk, prattle. GLOSSOLALIA – speaking in an unknown or imagined language in religious or other hysteria.
la(m)bda	G	A Greek letter, shaped so. LAMBDOID suture – the suture of the occipital and parietal skull bones.
lamina, lamella	L	A thin layer, usually of metal. LAMINECTOMY – removal of the vertebral arch.
lampros	G	Bright, splendid, distinct, sonorous. LAMPROPHONIA – clarity of speaking.
lanugo	L	Fine hairs, down. LANUGO – the downy hairs of a new-born infant.
lapara	G	Soft flank (of the belly). LAPAROTOMY – cutting open the abdomen.
lapaxy		See **alapazo.**
larynx; laryngos	G	The windpipe; pertaining to it. LARYNX.
lathyros	G	A kind of legume. LATHYRISM – illness from eating seeds of some leguminous plants.
latus	L	Side, or flank of the body. LATERAL.
lecithos	G	The yolk of eggs. LECITHIN – a phospholipid found in egg-yolk, and in many animal tissues.
leichon	G	Tree-moss, lichen, a blight. LICHEN
leios	G	Smooth, plain, unadorned. LEIOMYOMA – a benign tumour or fibroid, in the smooth muscle of the uterus.
leipo	G	To leave, desert, be wanting. LEIPOTHYMIA – syncope, faintness.

lemma	G	The outer layer, peel, skin. SARCOLEMMA – the membrane round a striped muscle fibre.
lemniscos	G	A ribbon, fillet, bandage. LEMNISCAL – pertaining to several bands of nervous tissue.
lenio	L	To assuage, soothe, mitigate. LENITIVE – soothing, demulcent.
lens, lentis	L	A lentil, shaped so. LENTICULAR – concerned with the eye lens or with lens-shaped structures.
lentigo	L	A freckle, a lentil-shaped spot. LENTIGINES – freckles. See lens.
lepros	G	Scaly, scabby, associated with leprosy and psoriasis. LEPROSY – a disease with granulomatous skin lesions.
lepsis	G	Seizing, catching. EPILEPSY – a paroxysmal disease due to abnormal brain activity.
leptos	G	Fine, delicate, narrow. LEPTOMENINGITIS – inflammation of the meninges of the central nervous system.
lepus; leporis	L	A hare; of it. LABIUM LEPORIS – hare-lip.
leucos, leukos	G	Clear, white. LEUCOCYTE – a white blood cell.
lexis	G	Speech, diction, words and phrases. DYSLEXIA – difficulty in understanding written language.
lien	L	The spleen. LIENOGASTRIC – concerned with the spleen and stomach.
ligo	L	To tie, bind. LIGATE.
limbus	L	An edge, border. LIMBIC – concerned with certain peripheral parts of the fore-brain.
limen	L	An entrance, doorway; LIMEN INFERUM – threshold. SUBLIMINAL – below the threshold of conscious appreciation.
limos	G	Hunger, famine. LIMOSIS – abnormal hunger.
linea	L	A linen thread; a stripe, line, mark. LINEA – a line, or linear mark.
lingua	L	A tongue. LINGUAL – pertaining to the tongue, glossal.
lino	L	To smear on, spread over. LINIMENT – a medical preparation rubbed on to the skin.
linon	G	Flax, linen, threads of linen. LINITIS – gastric in-

		flammation giving rise to fibrous tissue of a leathery texture.
lint		See **linon**.
lip, lipo		1. See **lipos**.
		2. See **leipo**.
lipos; liparos	G	Fat, tallow, oil; oily. LIPOPENIA – deficiency of body lipids.
lissos	G	Smooth. LISSENCEPHALIC – a brain without gyri.
lithos	G	Stone. LITHIASIS – disease with formation of stones or concretions.
locheia	G	Child-birth. LOCHIOCYTE – a cell characteristic of the vaginal discharge after childbirth.
loco		See **locus**.
loculus	L	A small chamber, box. MULTILOCULAR – having several chambers.
locus	L	A place. LOCUS – a particular place or defined region, often in the brain, e.g., LOCUS COERULEUS.
logas; logades	G	The eyeball, eyeballs; the whites of the eyes. LOGADITIS – inflammation of the sclera of the eye.
log, logo		See **logos**.
logos	G	A discourse, expression of thought. MORPHOLOGY – the study of form.
lophos	G	the nape of the neck, the crest of a bird; a ridge of hills. LOPHODONT – teeth with ridges.
lordos	G	Bent backwards. LORDOSIS – posterior concavity of the lumbar spine, "sway" or "saddle" back.
loxos	G	Oblique, slanting. LOXARTHRON – an oblique deformity of a joint.
luceo	L	To shine, be luminous. TRANSLUCENT – diffusely transmitting light.
luci		See **lux**.
lues	L	A plague, pestilence. LUETIC – syphilitic.
lumbricus	L	An intestinal worm; the earthworm. LUMBRICALES – small muscles of the hand and foot, thought to resemble small worms.
lumbus	L	The loin. LUMBAR.
lumen, luminis	L	1. Light, especially of a lamp, or from a window. LUMINOUS.

		2. A window, opening. LUMINAL – pertaining to the hollow of an organ.
luna	L	The moon. LUNATIC – a mentally deranged person, a state originally believed to be caused by the moon.
lunula	L	A cresent-shaped amulet. LUNULA – a crescent-shaped area, e.g., *lunula unguis*.
luo; lutum	L	To wash, cleanse; washed. ABLUTION – washing or cleaning with water.
lupus; lupinus	L	A wolf, something feared and destructive; pertaining to wolves. LUPUS – several types of ulcerous destructive diseases of the skin.
luteus	L	Yellow, reddish-yellow. CORPUS LUTEUM – an empty ovarian follicle containing yellow glandular tissue.
lux, lucis	L	Light, especially of the sun. LUCIFUGAL – avoiding bright light.
luxo	L	To dislocate. LUXATION – dislocation of a joint.
lycos	G	A "wolf" (originally probably a jackal). LYCANTHROPY – a delusion in which a person thinks he or she is a wolf.
lympha	L	Clear, spring water. LYMPHATIC – pertaining to lymph and the vessels containing this.
lyo	G	To loosen, unfasten, dissolve. LYSIS – breaking down of cells or tissues; freeing of an organ; abatement of a disease.
lyssa	G	Raging frenzy, furious madness. LYSSOPHOBIA – fear of rabies; or of having its symptoms.

M

macros	G	Large, long in time or space. MACROCYTE – an extra large red blood cell.
macula	L	A spot, blemish. MACULA LUTEA – a yellow depression in the retina, the "blind spot".
madao; madesis	G	To fall off, to be bald; loss of hair. ONYCHOMADESIS – total shedding of the nails.

magma	G	A thick unguent, a paste. MAGMA – a thin paste or suspension.
mala	L	The cheek bone, jaw bone, cheek. MALAR – pertaining to the cheek.
malacos	G	Soft, gentle, mild. OSTEOMALACIA – softening of the bones.
malignus	L	Malicious, injurious, wicked. MALIGNANT – virulent and becoming worse.
malleolus	L	A small hammer. MALLEOLUS – a rounded protuberance, e.g., that on the ankle.
malleus	L	A hammer. MALLEUS – one of the ear ossicles, roughly hammer-shaped.
mallos	G	A lock of wool. MALLOCHORION – a primitive mammalian chorion with many villi.
malus	L	Bad, abnormal. MALFUNCTION.
mamma	L	Breast. MAMMOGRAM – an X-ray picture of the mammary gland.
mammilla	L	A little breast, the nipple. MAMMELITIS – inflammation of the nipple. Cf. **thele.**
manos	G	Loose, thin, rare. MANOMETER – an instrument which measures fluid pressure.
manubrium	L	A shaft, handle. MANUBRIUM – the part of the sternum with which the first two pairs of ribs articulate.
manus	L	The hand. TALIPOMANUS – a hand deformation like club-foot.
margo	L	A border, edge, boundary. MARGO.
marisca	L	A haemorrhoid. MARISCAE – haemorrhoids.
maschale	G	The armpit, axilla. MASCHALONCUS – a tumour of the armpit.
masso	G	To knead, press into cakes. MASSOTHERAPY – treatment by massage. See **maza.**
mastichao	G	To gnash the teeth. MASTICATE.
mastiche	G	An aromatic gum used as chewing gum. MASTIC – a resinous substance used in dentistry and pharmaceutics.
mastos	G	The breast. MASTECTOMY – removal of a mammary gland. See **mazos.**

mater	L	Mother, a giver, producer. PIA MATER – the inner meninx.
maxilla	L	The (upper) jaw bone. MAXILLA.
maza	G	A small flat barley cake, shaped so. MAZIC – placental. See **masso**.
mazos	G	The breast. MAZOPLASIA – degenerative hypertrophy of mammary tissue. See **mastos**.
meatus	L	A passage, way, going. MEATUS – an opening. See also **meo**.
mecistos	G	Largest, longest. MECISTOCEPHALIC – having a head relatively long for its width. See **mecyno**.
mecon	G	The poppy, its juice. Also the intestinal contents of a new-born (perhaps because of similarity of colouring). MECONIUM.
mecos	G	Length, stature, distance. MECISM – abnormal length of a part.
mecyno	G	To lengthen, extend, prolong. MECYSTASIS – the property of some smooth muscles of having the same tension both before an imposed stretch and after returning to the original length.
medea	G	The genitalia. MEDORRHOEA – a discharge from the urethra.
medius	L	The middle. MEDIAN.
medulla	L	The marrow, pith, kernal, inmost part. MEDULLA – the innermost part of an organ.
megas, megala	G	Great, important. MEGAKARYOCYTE – a large bone-marrow cell from which platelets are derived.
meioo	G	To lessen, decrease. MEIOSIS – chromosomal reduction division.
melaena, melena		See **melas**.
melas; melanos	G	Black; of black. MELANIN – the dark brown pigment in various parts of the body.
meliceris	G	A honeycomb; a kind of cyst. MELICERA – a cyst filled with viscous fluid.
melon	G	An apple; shaped so; the cheek. MELONCUS – a tumour of the cheek.
melos	G	A limb. ANISOMELIA – a pair of unequal limbs.
mene	G	Month, moon. See **mensis**.

meninx	G	A membrane; the membrane around the brain. MENINGES – the membranes surrounding the central nervous system.
meniscos	G	A crescent. MENISCUS – a crescent-shaped structure, especially one of the cartilages on the proximal end of the tibia.
mens, mentis	L	The mind. MENTAL.
mensis	L	Month. DYSMENORRHOEA – painful menstruation.
mentula	L	The penis. MENTULAGRA – priapism.
mentum	L	The chin. MENTOLABIAL – relating to the chin and lips.
meo	L	To go, pass. PERMEABLE.
mephitis	L	A noxious vapour from the earth; malaria. MEPHITIC – emitting a foul stench.
meros	G	1. A part. METAMERE – a unit of a homologous series, especially in embryology. 2. The thigh. MEROCOXALGIA – pain in the thigh and hip.
mesio		See **mesos**.
mesos	G	The middle, mean, intermediate. MESODERM – the middle cell layer of an embryo lying between the ectoderm and endoderm.
met(a)	G	Between, among, along with, besides, behind. METASTASIS – the transfer of a disease to a site not adjacent to the original one, either by microorganisms or by tumour cells.
metachoresis	G	Departure, withdrawal. PHACOMETACHORESIS – displacement of the eye lens.
meter		See **metrios, metron**.
metopon	G	The space between the eyes, the forehead, front. METOPODYNIA – frontal headache.
metra	G	The uterus. ENDOMETRIUM – the uterine lining.
metrios, metron	G	Moderate, measure. DYSMETRIA – a form of ataxia in which accurate movement in relation to an object is lacking.
micros	G	Small, short. MICROSCOPE.
mictur		See **mingo**.
milium	L	Millet, its seed, shaped so. MILIARIA – a condition

in which there are skin lesions of a shape similar to millet seeds.

mimeticos	G	Able to imitate, imitative. SYMPATHOMIMETIC – used of drugs causing effects simulating sympathetic activity.
mingo; mictum	L	To urinate; urinated. MICTURITION – urinating.
mio		See **meioo**.
mistura		See **mixtura**.
mitos	G	A thread. MITOCHONDIRA – threadlike or granular organelles.
mitosis		A shortened form of **mitoschisis** (mito schisis) q.v.
mitto	L	To send away, release, emit. NEUROMITTOR – the element of the peripheral end of the presynaptic neurone releasing a transmitter substance.
mixtura	L	A mixture. MISTURA.
mnema, mneme	G	Memory, recollection, record. AMNESIA – loss of memory.
modiolus	L	The nave or hub of a wheel. MODIOLUS – the central pillar of the cochlear spiral.
mogis	G	With toil or pain; hardly. MOGIARTHRIA – defective speech articulation due to lack of muscle coordination.
mola	L	A mill-stone. MOLAR – a posterior grinding tooth.
mollis	L	Soft, tender, pliant. MOLLITIES – abnormal softening.
monas	G	Unitary, alone. MONOCYTE – a large phagocytic leucocyte.
monile	L	A necklace. MONILIFORM – like a string of beads.
morbidus	L	Sickly, unwholesome, diseased. MORBID.
morphe	G	Form, shape. MORPHOLOGY.
mors; mortis	L	Death; of it. POSTMORTEM – after death.
motor		See **moveo**.
moveo; motum	L	To move; moved. OCULOMOTOR – moving the eye.
mulceo	L	To soothe, allay pain. DEMULCENT – a substance which alleviates irritation or pain. (Better: mulcent.)
muliebris	L	Pertaining to women, feminine. MULIEBRIA – the female genitalia.

multus	L	Many. MULTICELLULAR – composed of many cells.
muto	L	To change, exchange. MUTAGENESIS – the process of (genetic) change.
mutus	L	Unable to speak, dumb. MUTISM.
my		See **mys**.
myces; mycetos	G	Fungus; of it. MYCOSIS – a disease caused by a fungus.
mycter	G	Nostril, snout. XEROMYCTERIA – dry mucous membranes in the nose
mydriasis	G	Dilation of the eye pupil. MYDRIASIS.
myelos	G	Marrrow; the brain, the spinal cord. MYELOCOEL – a hernia of the spinal cord through the spinal column.
myia	G	A fly, the bluebottle fly. MYIASIS – infection by fly maggots.
myle	G	A hand-mill, the lower millstone, the molar teeth. MYLOHYOID – of the muscle between the posterior part of the mandible and the hyoid bone. Cf. **mola**.
myo	G	1. To be shut, to close. MYOPIA – near sightedness. 2. See **mys**.
myringa	L?	The membrane of a drum. MYRINGOPLASTY – surgical repair of a perforated ear drum.
mys; myos	G	A muscle, a mouse; of these. MYOLOGY – the study of muscles of the body.
mysos	G	Uncleanliness, defilement. MYSOPHILIA – excitement from excretions, faeces, etc.
myxa	G	Slime, mucus. MYXOEDEMA – a disease involving deposits of mucin in the skin and other characteristic changes.

N

naevus	L	A mole (on the skin). NAEVUS – a stable deformity of a limited area of the skin.
nanos	G	A dwarf. NANOUS – dwarfish, stunted.
narce	G	Numbness, deadness, torpor. NARCOSIS – stupor, insensibility.

nascor; natus	L	To be born; born. ANTENATAL – concerned with the period before birth. PRENATAL.
nasus	L	The nose. NASOPHARYNX – appertaining to the nose and throat.
natis	L	A buttock. NATES – buttocks.
nato; natans	L	To swim, to float; floated. SUPERNATANT – the liquid phase after precipitation or centrifugation.
natrium, natrum		See **nitron**.
natus		See **nascor**.
nausia	G	Sea-sickness, nausea. NAUSEA – an unpleasant feeling often preceding vomiting.
necros	G	A corpse. NECROPSY – autopsy, examination of a corpse.
nema	G	A spun thread, yarn. TREPONEMA – a genus of sometimes spirally-formed parasitic microorganisms.
neos	G	New, young, youthful. NEOPLASM – new tissue; usually used to refer to uncontrolled growth.
nephros	G	The kidneys. NEPHRITIS – inflammation of the kidney.
nesos, nesidion	G	An islet, a little islet. NESIDIECTOMY – excision of the islets of Langerhans from the pancreas.
nestis	G	Fasting, starving. NESOTHERAPY – treatment by reduced intake of food.
neuron	G	1. A tendon, sinew. APONEUROSIS – the tough membrane in and around a skeletal muscle; also the extension of this connecting the muscle to a bone. 2. Also used for nerves. NEUROGENIC – producing nervous tissue; producing nervous excitation; produced by the nervous system.
nevus		See **naevus**.
nicto	L	To wink, blink. NICTITATION – winking.
nidus	L	A nest. NIDATION – implantation of the early embryo in the endometrium.
nisus	L	A straining; the pains of labour; an exertion. NISUS – effort, endeavour.

nitron	G	Sodium carbonate. Now related to the element sodium. NATRIURESIS – excess excretion of sodium in the urine.
noceo; noxa	L	To injure, hurt, harm; injurious action. NOCICEPTIVE – responsive to injurious stimuli.
nodus	L	A knot. NODE, NODULE, NODULUS – a small swelling.
noema	G	Something perceived, a thought, idea, purpose, understanding. Now implying without sensory perception. NOUMENON – something intuitively believed.
noesis	G	Intelligence, thought, cognition. NOESIS – cognition, rational thinking.
noia		See **noos** and **noesis**.
nome	G	Pasturage and grazing, spreading out; spreading sores and ulcers. NOMA – gangrenous sores of the mouth or genitalia.
nomos	G	Law, custom, convention. NOMOGRAM – a graphical representation of the relations beween several variables.
noos, nous	G	The mind, sense. PARANOIA – a personality disorder characterized by delusions of grandeur and irrational suspicions.
norma	L	A norm, standard. NORMOTHERMIC – having a normal temperature.
nosos	G	Disease, plague, anguish. NOSOLOGY – the classification of diseases.
nosteo	G	To return home. NOSTALGIA – longing to return home or to one's homeland.
noton, notos	G	The back. NOTOCHORD – the embryological midline structure lying ventral (anterior) to the neural tube, the precursor of the vertebrate spinal column.
nox; noctis	L	Night, darkness; of these. NOCTURIA – excessive urination at night.
noxi		See **noceo**.
nucleus	L	Kernal, stone of nut or fruit. NUCLEUS – the central organelle of a eukaryote cell. Also a collection

of nerve cells forming a subdivision within the nervous system.

nullus	L	None, not one. NULLIPAROUS – not having had a living child.
nuto	L	To nod the head, incline downwards; hesitate, waver. NUTATION – head nodding, usually involuntarily.
nycto		See **nyx**.
nyma		See **onoma, onyma**.
nymphe	G	A young woman, a bride, a nubile female. NYMPHOMANIAC – a woman with excessive sexual desire.
nysso	G	To prick, pierce, touch with a sharp point. HYALONYXIS – puncturing the vitreous body of the eye.
nystagmos	G	Drowsiness. NYSTAGMUS – involuntary rapid eye movements.
nyx; nyctos	G	1. Night; of it. NYCTOHEMERAL – circadian, pertaining to both day and night. 2. See **nysso** and cf. **nox**.

O

ob	L	A prefix indicating towards, at, against.
obduco	L	To cover, draw over. OBDUCTION – autopsy, postmortem examination.
obelos	G	A spit on which meat is speared; an obelisk. Now, like the vertex of an obelisk. OBELION – the point on the skull where a line joining the parietal foramina crosses the sagittal plane.
obex	L	A bolt, fastening, barrier. OBEX – a thickening of the ependyma at the inferior angle of the fourth ventricle of the brain.
obtundo; obtusum	L	To thump, make dull, blunt; deadened. OBTUDENT – a treatment with soothing medicine.
obturo	L	To stop up a hole, plug, block. OBTURATOR – a structure, natural or prosthetic, which closes an opening.

oc		See **ob**.
occludo	L	To close up, shut. OCCLUSION – a closure, of the teeth or of an opening
occultus	L	Hidden, obscure, secret. OCCULT – difficult to observe or understand.
ochlos	G	A throng, mob. OCHLOPHOBIA – a fear of crowds.
ochros	G	Pale, sallow, yellowish. OCHROMETER – a device for measuring capillary blood pressure, by applying pressure until blanching occurs.
oculus	L	The eye. OCULAR.
odax	G	Biting. ODAXEMUS – biting the tongue or cheek in an epileptic fit.
odont		See **odous**.
odous; odonticos	G	A tooth, spike, prong; dental. ODONTOLOGY – the study of dentition.
odyne	G	Pain, distress. ANODYNE – soothing, reducing pain.
oedema		See **oidema**.
oesophagus	G	The gullet. OESOPHAGUS, ESOPHAGUS.
oestrus		See **oistros**.
ogmos	G	A straight line, furrow, swathe. Now, an emission. ONEIROGMUS – emission of semen while asleep and dreaming.
ogogue		See **agogue**.
oicos	G	A house, home, abode. ECOLOGY (OECOLOGY) – the study of biological communities.
oid		See **eidos**.
oidema	G	Swelling, tumour. OEDEMA – excessive tissue fluid, often subcutaneous.
oistros	G	A gadfly, a sting of pain; an insane passion. OESTRUS – the period of sexual activity in non-hominid mammals.
olecranon	G	The point of the elbow. OLECRANON – This word might be "OLENOCRANION" from **olene** and **cranion**, q.v.
olene	G	The ulna, the lower arm. ULNA.
oleum	G	Oil. OLEORESIN – a mixture of oil and resin.
olfacio	L	To smell. OLFACTOMETER – an instrument used to measure olfactory sensitivity.

oligakis	G	Seldom. OLIGAKISURIA – urinating relatively seldom.
oligos	G	Small, few. OLIGOSPERMIA – having semen with a low sperm count.
olisthano	G	To slip. SPONDYLOLISTHESIS – forward displacement of a vertebra.
oma	G	A suffix indication a tumour or other abnormal growth, perhaps derived from **oncos**, q.v. CARCINOMA – a cancerous tumour.
omentum	L	The embryonic caul; also the bowels. OMENTUM – the peritoneal membrane holding the viscera in the abdominal cavity.
omos	G	1. The shoulder and upper arm. ACROMION – the projection on the scapula at the shoulder. 2. Raw, unripe, coarse. OMOPHAGIA – the eating of raw food.
omphalos	G	A round boss or button; the stone marking the centre of the world; the navel. OMPHALITIS – inflammation of the navel.
oncos	G	1. A large mass, bulk, weight. ONCOLOGY – the study of tumours. 2. A barb on an arrow. ONCOSPHERE – one of the larval stages of a tapeworm with an involuted head on which are hooks.
oncus		See **oncos**.
oneiros	G	A dream. ONEIRANALYSIS – analysis of pharmacologically induced dreams.
onoma, onyma	G	Name. ANOMIA – inability to name objects.
onyx; onycho	G	A nail, claw; of these. PARONYCHIA – disease of the skin folds around the nails.
oon	G	An egg. OOCYTES – female reproductive cells undergoing the last two stages in their maturation to ova. See **ovum**.
ophis	G	A snake, serpent. OPHIOTOXAEMIA – snake venom poisoning.
ophrys	G	The brow, eyebrow. OPHRYON – the middle point between the eyebrows.
ophthalmos	G	The eye. OPHTHALMOLOGY – the study of the eye.

opia		See **opsis**.
opisthen	G	After, behind, rear, back. OPISTHOTONUS – a spasm with excessive tension in the back musculature.
ops	G	Face. OPSALGIA – neuralgia of the face. Cf. **opse**.
opse	G	After a long time; late, in the evening. OPSIURIA – increased urine production during fasting.
opsi		See **opse** or **opsis**.
opsis	G	Appearance, countenance, the eye. ACHROMATOPSIA – total colour blindness. Cf. **ops**.
opson	G	Prepared victuals, provisions, cooked meats. OPSONIN – a substance which makes bacteria more susceptible to phagocytosis.
opticos	G	Concerned with the laws of optics. OPTICIAN. See also **opsis**.
or, oro		See **oros** or **os**.
orbis; orbitus	L	A ring or circle; circular. ORBITA – the eye socket.
orchis	G	The testicle or ovary. ORCHIDECTOMY – removal of a testis.
orexis	G	Appetite, desire. ANOREXIA – lack of desire to eat.
orizo	G	To separate, divide from, delimit. HYPERTELORISM – abnormally large distance between two organs, e.g., the eyes.
oros	G	Serum. ORORRHOEA – a serous discharge.
orrhos		See **oros**.
orthos	G	Straight, correct, upright. ORTHODONTICS – the treatment of irregularities of teeth development.
orthrios	G	Daybreak, early in the morning. ORTHRIOPSIA – having maximum visual acuity in relatively poor light.
os; oris	L	The mouth, oral. ORAL.
os, osseum	L	A bone; made of bone. OSSEOFIBROUS – made of a mixture of bone and fibrous tissue.
osche	G	The scrotum. OSCHEONCUS – a scrotal tumour.
oscito	L	To open the mouth, gape, yawn. OSCITATION – yawning.

osis	G	A suffix meaning a condition, process, activity. TUBERCULOSIS – a disease in which there is tubercle formation. See also **iasis**.
osme, osmos	G	1. Odour, smell, scent. ANOSMIA – inability to smell. See also **osphresis**. 2. Thrust, attack. OSMOSIS – movement of solvent, but not solute, from a less to a more concentrated solution, through a semi-permeable membrane.
osphresis	G	The sense of smell. OSPHRESIS. See also **osme**.
osphys	G	The loins, lower part of the back. OSPHYARTHROSIS – inflammation of the hip joint.
osseo	L	See **os, osseum**.
osteon	G	Bone. OSTEOBLAST – a cell intimately concerned with the formation of bone.
ostium	L	A door, an entrance. OSTIUM.
ot, otic		See **ous**.
oule	G	The scar of a wound, a cicatrix. EPULOSIS – formation of new tissue, scarring.
oulon	G	The gums of the teeth. ULORRHOEA – bleeding from the gums.
ourachos	G	The urachus. URACHUS.
ouranos; ouraniscos	G	A vault, the heavens; shaped so. Now, the vault of the mouth, the palate. URANISCOCHASMA – a cleft palate.
oureo	G	To pass water. DIURESIS – passing a large volume of urine.
ouron	G	Urine. URAEMIA – excess urea, and similar nitrogneous waste products, in the blood.
ous; otis	G	The ear, a jug handle, the auricles of the heart; of these. OTITIS – ear inflammation.
ovum	L	An egg. OVULATION – the release of an egg from the ovary.
oxyno	G	To make acute, make acid, sharpen. PAROXYSM – a sudden seizure or a sudden increase in the severity of symptoms.
oxys	G	Sharp, acute. OXYTOCIC – a substance or procedure promoting uterine contractions.

| ozaina | G | A foetid polypus in the nose. OZAEMA – a thick, foetid discharge from the nose. |
| ozo | G | To smell. OZOSTOMIA – foul smell from the mouth. |

P

pachys	G	Thick, very large, coarse. PACHYBLEPHARON – thickening of the eyelids.
paed		See **pais**.
paedeuo		See **paideuo**.
pag, pagus		See **pagos** and **pegnymi**.
pagos	G	Fixed, coagulated, ice, frost. PAGOPLEXIA – frostbite.
paideuo	G	To teach, educate. PROPAEDEUTIC – concerned with preliminary instruction, introductory teaching.
pais, paidos	G	A child, slave. PAEDIATRICS – the study of children's diseases and malfunctions.
palaios	G	Ancient, venerable, obsolete. PALEOPALLIUM – part of the cerebrum which has evolved from the olfactory region of the primitive vertebrate brain.
palin	G	Back again, backwards, contradiction. PALILALIA – frequent repetition of a word or phrase.
palla	L	A wide cloak. PALLIUM – the cerebral cortex and its developmental precursor.
pallidus	L	Pale in colour. PALLIDOTOMY – the making of lesions in the globus pallidus.
pallo	G	To shake, sway, swing, quiver, leap. PALLAESTHESIA – vibration sensitivity, especially to that received via the bones.
palpate		See **palpo**.
palpebra	L	The eyelid. PALPEBRAL fissure – the opening between the eyelids.
palpito	L	To beat, move quickly, frequently. PALPITATION – heart beat felt by a person in his or her own chest.
palpo	L	To touch or stroke gently. PALPATION – feeling with the hand or fingers.

pampinus	L	A (vine-)tendril. PAMPINIFORM – applied to a complex of veins adjacent to the testis or ovary.
pan; panta		See **pas.**
pannus; **panniculus**	L	A piece of cloth, rag, bandage; a little garment. PANNICULUS – a thin layer of tissue clearly different from adjacent tissues.
papilla	L	A small nipple. PAPILLA – any small nipple-shaped process or projection.
papula	L	A pimple, pustule. PAPULA – a firm elevated lesion up to about one centimeter in diameter.
par(a)		1. Alongside, resembling, far beyond. PARAMEDIAN – near the midline. 2. Faulty. PARAMNESIA – faulty remembrance or inability to understand remembered words.
paresis	G	A letting go, paralysis, slackening of strength. PARESIS – some degree of paralysis. See also **hiemi.**
paric		See **pario.**
paries	L	A wall, an enclosing structure. PARIETAL – related to the walls of a hollow structure.
pario; partum	L	To bring forth; born. NULLIPAROUS – not having borne a living child.
parvus	L	Small. PARVOVIRUS – a small virus.
pas, pan	G	All. PANDEMIC – a disease affecting the majority of the people of the world.
patens	L	Open. PATENT.
pathos; **patheticos**	G	Suffering, emotion; of sensation. PATHOLOGY – the study of disease.
patulus	L	Open, expanded. PATULOUS – widely open.
pechys	G	The fore-arm, the ulna, its length. PECHYAGRA – gout in the elbow.
pecten	L	A comb, rake. PECTENITIS – inflammation of the comb-like fold in the anal canal.
pectos	G	Curdled, congealed, fixed. PECTIN – a polysaccharide which forms gels with sucrose.
pectus; pectoris	L	The breast; pectoral. PECTORAL – pertaining to the chest or breast.
ped		See **pes.**
pedao; pedesis	G	To leap, throb; leaping flames over a fire.

DIAPEDESIS – a mistaken spelling for DIAPEIRESIS. See **peiro.**

pedem		See **pedao.**
pedesis		See **peiro.**
pediculus	L	A little foot, a pedicle; a louse. PEDICLE – a stalk.
pegnymi	G	To make fast, fasten together. THORACOPAGUS – a twin monster united anteriorly at the thorax.
peiro	G	To pierce through. DIAPEIRESIS – the passage of cells from the blood through the vessel walls.
pella	G	A wooden bowl, shaped so. LEPTOPELLA – a narrow pelvis.
pellis	L	The skin. PELLAGRA – a disease in which there is dermatitis, due to lack of niacin.
pello; pulsus	L	To strike, knock against; a blow. PULSE – the pressure wave in an artery which can be felt with the fingers.
pelos	G	Clay, mud, mire. PELOHAEMIA – excess viscosity of the blood.
pelvis	L	A basin. PELVIS.
pemphigodes	G	With vesicular eruptions. PEMPHIGUS – designates diseases characterized by many bullae or large vesicles.
penia	G	Lack, poverty. CYTOPENIA – a lack of blood cells.
penna	L	A feather, constructed so; a wing. BIPENNIFORM – a rachis with bilateral branches, each of which is also built on the same pattern. Often wrongly used of muscles which are penniform, not bipenniform. See also **pinna.**
pente	G	Five. PENTOSE – a sugar molecule containing five carbon atoms.
peos	G	The penis. PEOECTOMY – removal of the penis.
pepsis	G	Ripening, cooking, softening of food. PEPSIN – the proteolytic enzyme in gastric juice. See **pesso.**
per	L	1. Through, via. PERCEPTION – the mental appreciation of stimuli. 2. Indicates emphasis, more of something. PERTUSSIS – a severe cough, whooping cough.
peral		See **pario.**

peri	G	Near, around. PERIOSTEUM – the layers of connective tissue covering the bones.
perineos	G	The region between the anus and the genitalia. PERINEUM.
peritonaios	G	A stretched covering, especially that covering the abdominal viscera. PERITONEUM.
permeable		See **meo**.
perniones	L	Chilblains of the feet. PERNIO – a chillblain of the foot.
perone	G	A piercing object, a pin, the fibula. PERONEAL – pertaining to the fibula. Cf. **fibula**.
peros	G	Maimed. PEROMELIA – congenital deformity of a limb.
pes; pedis	L	The foot; of it. PEDOMETER – an instrument measuring the number of steps in walking.
pesso	G	To ripen, cook, digest. PEPTIC – related to pepsin, gastric juice and stomach activity. See **pepsis**.
petechia	I	A small skin extravasation. PETECHIAE.
peto	L	To attack, aim at, strive towards. LUCIPETAL – seeking or moving towards a bright light.
petros	G	Stone. OSTEOPETROSIS – with excessively dense bones.
pexis	G	Fixation, coagulation. NEPHROPEXY – the surgical fastening of a loose kidney. See **pegnymi**.
phacos	G	A lentil, shaped so. PHACOSCLEROSIS – hardening of the eye lens.
phagein	G	To eat, devour. PHAGOCYTOSIS – ingestion by cells.
phaino	G	To make known, reveal, make clear, shine out. CHROMOPHANE – a pigment of the retina.
phaios	G	Dusky, grey. HAEMAPHEIN – a brown substance colouring blood and urine.
phakos		See **phacos**.
phalanx	G	The line of a battle array; a round piece of wood, shaped so. PHALANGES – the units of the digits.
phallos	G	The penis, symbol of generation. PHALLUS.
phaneros	G	Visible, manifest, evident. PHANEROGENIC – hav-

		ing a known cause; opposite to cryptogenic. See **phaino**.
pharmacon	G	A drug, poison, remedy. PHARMACOLOGY – the study of drugs.
pharynx	G	The throat, windpipe. PHARYNX – the upper extremity of the gullet.
phasis	G	Statement, rumour. DYSPHASIA – impaired, uncoordinated speech.
phein		See **phaios**.
phemia	G	Utterance, prophecy. DYSPHEMIA – stuttering, disordered speech.
phen		See **phaino**. PHENOMENON.
phero	G	To bear, carry. PERIPHERY – the outer edge or surface of a structure. See **phoreo** and **fero**.
phileo	G	To love, to treat affectionately. BASOPHIL – of cells or tissues staining well with basic dyes.
philtron	G	The median groove of the upper lip. PHILTRUM.
phimosis	G	Muzzling; contraction of the prepuce. PHIMOSIS – a strangulating foreskin preventing its retraction.
phleb		See **phleps**.
phlegma	G	Inflammation, heat, a morbid humour. PHLEGM – excessive, viscid mucus, especially from the respiratory tract.
phlego	G	To burn, inflame. ADENOPHLEGMON – inflammation of the stroma of a gland. Cf. **phlox**.
phleps; phlebos	G	A blood vessel; of this. PHLEBITIS – inflammation of veins.
phlog		See **phlego, phlox**.
phlox; phlogos	G	A flame; of it. PHLOGOCYTE – a plasma cell typically found in inflamed tissue. See **phlego**.
phlyctaina	G	A blister. PHLYCTENULE – a small vesicle or ulcer on the cornea or conjutiva.
phlysis	G	An eruption. GALACTOPHLYSIS – a vesicle containing a milky fluid.
phobos	G	Panic, terror. PHOBIA – irrational, morbid fear.
phoce	G	A seal (sea mammal). PHOCOMELIA – a monster having the limbs reduced to small appendages.

phone	G	The voice, a sound. PHONOGRAM – a recording of sound.
phoreo	G	To bear, carry constantly, wear, to be carried away. OOPHORON – the ovary. See also **phero** and **fero**.
phos; photos	G	Light; of it. PHOTOPHOBIA – intolerance and dislike of light.
photo		See **phos**.
phragma		See **phrax**, and **phrasso**.
phrasis	G	Speech, expression. PALIPHRASIA – inordinate repetition of words or phrases.
phrasso	G	To fence in, to block up, make close. EMPHRAXIS – a stoppage or obstruction. See **phrax**.
phrax, phragma	G	1. A fence. DIAPHRAGM – the transverse muscular layer between the thorax and the abdomen. 2. See **phrasso**.
phren	G	1. The midriff. Also the heart, the seat of the emotions. PHRENOPLEGIA – paralysis of the diaphragm. Cf. **thymos**. 2. The mind. SCHIZOPHRENIA – a mental disease with delusions and other effects.
phrictos	G	To be shuddered at, horrible. PHRICTOPATHIC – of a peculiar sensation during recovery from an hysterical episode.
phryne	G	A toad. PHRYNOLYSIN – the venom of the fire-toad *Bombinator igneus*.
phthisis	G	Decay, wasting away. PHTHISIS – wasting, especially in tuberculosis.
phthongos	G	A clear sound, vocal or musical. HETEROPHTHONGIA – speech anomaly.
phycos	G	Seaweed; orchil: a red or violet rouge prepared from seaweed. Now related to other algae and to fungi. PHYCOMYCOSIS – infection with fungi of the genus *Phycomycetes*.
phyge	G	Flight, escape, exile. GALACTOPHYGOUS – stopping milk secretion.
phylactic		See **phylaxis**.
phylaxis	G	Guarding. PROPHYLAXIS – preventive treatment.

phyle	G	A tribe, race, clan. MONOPHYLECTIC – derived from one cell type.
phyma	G	A tumour, swelling, growth. RHINOPHYMA – swelling and sebaceous hyperplasia of the skin of and around the nose.
phyo	G	To produce, beget, acquire, grow. See **physis**.
physallis	G	Bladder, bubble. PHYSALLIPHOROUS – containing bubbles or vesicles. Cf. **pompholyx**.
physema	G	A breath, blast, snort. EMPHYSEMA – abnormal interstitial gas or air, especially in the lungs.
physis	G	1. Origin, growth. EPIPHYSES – secondary centres of bone formation at the ends or margins of bones. See **phyo**. 2. The nature of something, natural order. PHYSIOLOGY – the study of the functioning of organisms.
phyton	G	A plant. DERMATOPHYTE – a skin fungus.
pia mater	A,L	The tender mother. PIA MATER – the inner meninx.
pies		See **piezo**.
piezo	G	To press, squeeze. AEROPIEZOTHERAPY – therapy involving air at greater or less than atmospheric pressure.
pilos	G	Felted wool or hair. PILOERECTOR – muscles causing erection of the hairs.
pimele	G	Soft fat, lard. PIMELOMA – a fatty tumour.
pinguis	L	Fat. PINGUICULA – a yellowish spot near the sclerocorneal junction of the eye, usually on the nasal side and in elderly people.
pinna	L	A wing, feather. PINNA – the external part of the ear. See also **penna**.
pino	G	To drink. PINOCYTOSIS – ingestion of liquid by cellular invaginations.
pion	G	Fat, rich milk. PIONAEMIA – fat or oil in the blood.
pirum	L	A pear. PIRIFORM – pear-shaped.
pisum	L	A pea. PISIFORM – pea-shaped.
pithecos	G	An ape, monkey. PITHECANTHROPOID – like apes and mankind.
pituita	L	Rheum, slime, phlegm. PITUITARY – the endocrine

gland beneath the brain (formerly thought to produce the nasal mucus).

pityron   G   Bran, dandruff. PITYRIASIS – a group of skin diseases which entail different kinds of desquamation.

placenta   L   A thin, flat cake. PLACENTA – the foetal-maternal connection, which in humans is cake-shaped.

placeo   L   To please, be agreeable. PLACEBO – something given to please a patient, but without other known physiological effect.

plagios   G   Aslant, oblique, crooked. PLAGIOCEPHALY – an asymmetry of the cranium.

planos   G   Deceiving, fickle. MENOPLANIA – abnormal menses.

planta   L   The sole of the foot. PLANTIGRADE – using the whole of the foot when walking.

plasia   See **plasso**.

plasma   G   That which is moulded or formed. PLASMA. See **plasso**.

plasso   G   To form, mould. THORACOPLASTY – removal of ribs to produce and maintain a collapsed lung.

platys   G   Broad, flat. PLATYRRHINE – with a flattened nose.

plax; plakous   G   Flat and broad; of a flat cake like a melon seed. LEUKOPLAKIA – whitish patches on mucous membranes, mainly of the mouth.

plectron   G   A striking instrument or tool. PLECTRON – the hammer shape of certain bacterial spores.

plege   G   A stroke, blow, an impact. HEMIPLEGIA – unilateral paralysis of the body.

pleion, pleon   G   More, plus, greater. PLEIONECTIC – blood more saturated than normal at a given tension of oxygen.

plesios   G   Near, close to. PLESIOMORPHIC – having nearly the same form.

plesso   G   To hit, smite. PLEXIMETER – a glass plate interposed between finger and skin in percussion and the application of pressure.

plethyo   G   To become full, swell, increase. PLETHYSMOGRAPH

		– an apparatus to show changes in the volume of body structures enclosed within it.
pleuron	G	A rib, the side of the body. PLEURAL.
plex		See **plexus** or **plesso**.
plexus	L	Twisted, plaited, twined, braided. PLEXUS.
plico	L	To fold, fold together. PLICATE.
pneuma	G	Air, breath, breathing; the spirit, soul. PNEUMOTHORAX – the presence of air in the pleural cavity.
pneumon	G	The lung, the organ of breathing. PNEUMONOPATHY – disease of the lungs.
pnoeo	G	A breath, blast, exhalation. APNOEA – absence of breathing.
pogon	G	The beard. POGONIASIS – excessive growth of beard; growth of a beard on a woman.
pod		See **pous**.
poiesis	G	Production, creation. HAEMOPOIETIC – forming blood.
poikilos	G	Of many different colours, diversified, changeable. POIKILOTHERMIC – of animals whose temperature largely varies with the environmental temperature.
poleo	G	To go about, range over, haunt. PERIPOLESIS – the clustering of lymphocytes around macrophages.
polios	G	Grey, hoary, grey-haired. POLIOMYELITIS – a disease with various symptoms and signs, sometimes involving the grey matter of the spinal cord.
pollakis	G	Often, many, mostly, altogether. POLLAKIDIPSIA – feeling thirsty very often.
polys	G	Many, much, often, great. POLYDACTYLY – having extra digits.
pompholyx	G	A blister. CHEIROPOMPHOLYX – a skin disease with vesicles deep under the skin of the hands and feet.
pomum	L	Fruit. POMUM ADAMI – the adam's apple.
ponos	G	Toil, suffering, grief, pain. PONOGRAPH – an instrument for measuring sensitivity to pain.
pons; pontis	L	A bridge; of it. PONTOCEREBELLAR – pertaining to the pons and cerebellum.

poples; poplitis	L	The ham, hough; of the back of the knee. POPLITEAL – pertaining to the knee.
poroo	G	To become calloused, hard. POROCELE – scrotal hernia, with thick, hard scrotal skin. Sometimes called porocoel.
poros	G	A narrow passage or hole. Later used to mean porous. OSTEOPOROSIS – demineralization of the bones, rarefaction of the skeleton.
porosis	G	Reunion of fractured bones by a callus. POROSIS. Cf. **poroo**.
porphyra	G	A red-brown purplish dye from the fish *Murex*. PORPHYRIA – disease with increased secretion of porphyrins, staining the urine. See also **purpura**.
porta	L	A gate, entrance. PORTA HEPATIS – the place where vessels and ducts enter and leave the liver.
posis	G	A drink drinking. ANTIPOSIS – antipathy to drinking.
posterus	L	Subsequent, following. POSTGANGLIONIC – distal to a ganglion.
posthe, posthia	G	The prepuce. POSTHITIS – inflammation of the prepuce.
pous; podis	G	The foot; of this. PODIATRIST – one who treats foot dysfunctions and diseases. Cf. **chiropodist**.
prae	L	Before. PRECURSOR – that which occurs first and foreshadows subsequent events.
pragma	G	A deed, event, affair. PRAGMATIC – concerned with events, their causes and their consequences.
prandium	L	The midday meal, any meal. POSTPRANDIAL – after a meal.
praxis	G	Doing something, activity. NEURAPRAXIA – paralysis, usually temporary, after an insult to a nerve. Cf. **neurotmesis**.
pre		See **prae**.
presbys	G	An old man. PRESBYOPIA – long sight in old age.
Priapos	G	The god of procreation; the penis. PRIAPISM – penile erection without respite.
primus	L	First. PRIMIGRAVIDA – a woman pregnant for the first time.

prio; prisis	G	To saw; sawing, trephining, grinding. ODONTOPRISIS – grinding of the teeth, especially when asleep.
pro	G	Forward, at the front of. PRODROMAL – precursal, premonitory.
proctos	G	The anus. PROCTODERM – the invaginated ectoderm forming the posterior end of the embryological gut.
prolabor; prolapsus	L	To slip forwards, slip out; fallen. PROLAPSE.
proles	L	Offspring. PROLIGERUS – producing offspring.
pronus	L	Bent forwards, stooping, inclined. PRONATE – with the palms facing down or posteriorly; lying face-down. Opposite to supine.
proprius	L	One's own, special. PROPRIOCEPTORS – receptors for monitoring body position and movement.
pros	G	From, from the side of, towards. PROSENCEPHALON – the embryological forebrain.
prosopon	G	The face, appearance. DIPROSOPUS – monster with at least partly two faces.
prosthesis	G	An addition, supplement, appendage. PROSTHETICS – learning concerned with prostheses.
prostates	G	One who stands before. The prostate gland. PROSTATE. See statos.
proteios	G	Of first quality. PROTEIN. See protos.
protos	G	First of all others, the very first. PROTOPLASM, PROTEIN.
prurio	L	To itch. PRURIGO – itchy skin lesions. Cf. psora.
psammos	G	Sand. PSAMMOMA – a tumour containing granular matter, psammoma bodies.
psathyros	G	Friable. ANGIOPSATHRYROSIS – abnormal fragility of blood vessels.
pselaphesis	G	Feeling, touching, palpation. PSELAPHESIA – the sense of touch.
pseudes	G	A falsehood. PSEUDOANGINA – symptoms simulating angina in nervous people.
psittacos	G	A parrot. PSITTACOSIS – a disease transmittable to

humans, first noted from parrots. Occurs also in other birds.

psoa	G	The muscles of the loins. PSOAS – muscles from the spine to the pelvic girdle and femur.
psomos	G	Gobbet, morsel. PSOMOPHAGIA – eating food without chewing it.
psora	G	An itch, mange, scab. PSORIASIS – a dermatosis with distinctive itching lesions. Cf. **prurio**.
psyche	G	Soul, life, conscious self. PSYCHOANALYSIS – therapeutic examination of the personality.
psychros	G	Cold. PSYCHROALGIA – painful feeling from being cold.
ptenos	G	Flying, winged, fleeting. Now, volatile. ELEOPTEN – the volatile fraction of an oil.
pteryx; pterygotos	G	A wing; of a wing. PTERION – the junction of the wing of the sphenoid with the frontal, parietal and temporal bones.
ptoma	G	A fallen man, a corpse, carcass, misfortune, calamity. PTOMAINE – a bacterial toxin. See also **ptosis**.
ptosis	G	A fall, falling. BLEPHAROPTOSIS – a drooping eyelid. See also **ptoma**.
ptyalin		See **ptyo**.
ptych		See **ptyx**.
ptyo	G	To spit out, to spit up. HAEMOPTYSIS – expectoration of blood or bloody mucus.
ptyx, ptyche	G	A fold, leaf, plate. ENTEROPTYCHIS – folding of the intestine to hinder the formation of adhesions.
pubes	L	1. Adult. PUBERTY – the period during which a person becomes sexually mature. 2. The pubic region; the growth of hair associated with puberty. PUBIC.
pubesco	L	To become adult, at the age of puberty. PUBESCENT – coming to the age of puberty, or having a covering of fine hairs.
pubis		See **pubes**.
pudendus	L	Shameful, disgraceful. PUDENDAL – concerned with the female genital region.

puer	L	A (young) boy, a child. PUERPERAL – pertaining to the period immediately after parturition.
pulex; pulicis	L	A flea; of a flea. PULICIDE – an agent which kills fleas.
pulmo; pulmonis	L	A lung; of it. PULMONARY.
pulsus		See **pello**.
pulvinus	L	A cushion, pillow. PULVINUS – a part of the thalamus resembling a cushion.
punctum	L	A little hole, spot or point. PUNCTIFORM – shaped like a dot.
purgo	L	To cleanse, clean out. PURGATION – evacuation of the bowels by cathartic medicine.
purpura	L	The purple dye, purple, violet. PURPURA – bruises and petechiae; subepidermal haemorrhages, giving bluish or dark red patches. See also **porphyra**.
purulentus	L	Containing much pus, exuding pus. PURULENT – pus forming, containing or caused by pus.
pus; puris	L	1. The purulent matter formed in an inflamed region. PUS. 2. See **pyon**.
pustula	L	A small swelling, pimple. PUSTULE – limited skin elevations containing pus.
putamen	L	A paring, shell, peel. PUTAMEN – the outer part of the lenticular nucleus of the brain.
py		See **pyon**.
pycnos		See **pyknos**.
pyelos	G	A trough, vat, shaped so. PYELITIS – inflammation of the kidney pelvis.
pyge	G	The rump, buttocks. STEATOPYGIA – excessively fat buttocks especially in women.
pyknos	G	Dense, thick, stocky, crowded. PYKNOMETER – an hydrometer.
pyle	G	One of a pair of double gates. PYLEPHLEBITIS – inflammation of the portal vein.
pyloros	G	A gate-keeper. PYLORUS – the opening between stomach and duodenum.
pyon	G	Pus. PYOMETRA – a purulent discharge from the uterus.

pyr	G	Fire, flame, fever heat. PYROGEN – a substance which produces fever.
pyren	G	The stone or kernal of fruits. PYRENAEMIA – presence of blood with nucleated red cells.
pyresso	G	To be feverish. PYREXIA – a fever.
pyreto, pyrexis		See **pyresso**.

Q

quadri		A combining form from **quattuor**, q.v. CORPORA QUADRIGEMINA – two double small swellings of the mid-brain.
quattuor	L	Four. QUADRIPLEGIA – paralysis of all four limbs. Cf. **tetraplegia**.
quintus	L	Fifth. DIGITUS QUINTUS – the little finger.

R

racemus	L	A cluster, especially of grapes, shaped so. RACEMOSE.
radior; radiatus	L	To gleam, shine, radiate; having rays. RADIOACTIVE – giving off corpuscular or electromagnetic radiation.
radius	L	A ray, spoke of a wheel, rod, stake, a bone of the fore-arm. RADIOULNAR – pertaining to the radius and ulna bones.
radix; radicis	L	A root; of it. RADICULITIS – inflammation of spinal nerve roots.
râle	F	The death-rattle. RALES – now also abnormal sounds in the lungs. Cf. **rhonchos**.
ramus	L	A branch. RAMI – the subdivisions of branching structures.
rarus	L	Uncommon, wide apart, opposite to dense. RAREFACTION – the state of becoming or being less dense.
re	L	A prefix indicating repetition. RESTENOSIS – recurrent stenosis.

recipio	L	To receive, take back. RECEPTOR – an organ responsive to certain stimuli.
rectus	L	Straight, correct. RECTUM – the short, straight part of the hindgut.
renes	L	The kidneys. SUPRARENAL.
restis	L	A rope. RESTIFORM – long and narrow, ropelike.
retro	L	Backwards, behind. RETROGRADE – progressing in a direction opposite to normal; or opposite to anterograde.
rhabdos	G	A wand, stick, staff. RHABDOVIRUS – a short, stubby virus.
rhachis	G	The spine, any ridge-shaped structure. RHACHIALGIA – pain in the spinal column.
rhagas	G	A chink, fissure. RHAGADES – fine cracks in the skin, especially near the mouth.
rhage		See **rhegnymi.**
rhaphe	G	A seam, suture. COLPORRHAPHY – narrowing of the vagina by a longitudinal line of sutures.
rhegnymi, rhegnuo	G	To break asunder, to let loose. HAEMORRHAGE – bleeding, loss of blood.
rheo; rhoia	G	To flow, run, pour; flux. DIARRHOEA – passing frequent and/or excessive, faeces.
rheuma	G	A flow, stream, flux. RHEUMATISM – originally, a disease associated with a rheumy, catarrhal discharge.
rhexis	G	A bursting apart, a tear. GASTRORHEXIS – rupture of the stomach. From **rhegnymi,** q.v.
rhis, rhinos	G	The nose; nasal. RHINITIS – inflammation of the nasal mucus membranes.
rhiza	G	A root. RHIZOTOMY – cutting spinal nerve roots within the spinal canal.
rhodon, rhodoeis	G	Rose, of roses; rose-coloured. RHODOPSIN – the purplish-red visual pigment in the retina.
rhoia, rhoid		See **rheo.**
rhonchos, rhonchmos	G	Wheezing. RHONCHUS – rattling in the throat or chest. Cf. rales.
rhypos	G	Filth. RHYPIA – thick skin crusts seen in late secondary syphilis. Often wrongly spelled rupia.

rhytis	G	A fold or pucker in the face. RHYTIDECTOMY – eliminating wrinkles by removal of skin. Cf. **ruga**.
rictus	L	The opening of the mouth, the gape. RICTUS.
rima	L	A cleft, crack, fissure. RIMA ORIS – the mouth aperture.
risus	L	Laughter. RISUS – an involuntary grimace from spasm of the facial muscles.
rostrum	L	The beak of snout of a bird or other animal. ROSTRAD – towards the head end.
ruber, rubor	L	Red. RUBEFACIENT – causing reddening hyperaemia of the skin.
rubellus	L	See **ruber**. RUBELLA – measles with pink skin eruptions.
ruga	L	A wrinkle in the face. RUGAE. Cf. **rhytis**.
rupia	L	See **rhypos**.

S

sacchar, saccharon	G	Sugar. POLYSACCHARIDE – a carbohydrate formed from many sugar molecules.
saccus, sacculus	L	A sac, a little sac. SAC.
sacer; sacrum	L	Holy; a sacred thing. SACRUM – the lower part of the spine, inferior to the lumbar region. Cf. **hieros**.
saeptum	L	A barrier, wall, enclosure. SEPTUM – a dividing layer or structure.
saeta	L	A stiff hair or bristle. SETIFEROUS – bearing bristles.
sagitta	L	An arrow. SAGITTAL – pertaining to the medial suture of the skull; also, planes parallel to the medial plane of the body.
salpinx; salpingos	G	A war trumpet; of this. SALPINGITIS – inflammation of the uterine or auditory tubes (shaped like trumpets).
saltatio	L	A dance, dancing. SALTATORY – leaping, jumping.
sanguis; sanguinis	L	Blood; bloody. SANGUINEOUS – full of blood.

sanies	L	Foetid bloody matter, pus, a discharge. SANIES – foetid purulent bloody discharge from a wound or ulcer.
saphes	G	Plain, obvious. SAPHENOUS – of the two large, obvious veins of the leg.
sapo	L	Soap. SAPONINS – plant substances which foam with water and lyse red blood cells.
sapros	G	Putrid, rotten. SAPRAEMIA – septic blood from infection with putrefying organisms.
sarcina	L	A bundle. SARCINA – bacteria which are usually found in groups of eight.
sarcio; sartum	L	To mend or repair, patch clothes; mended. SARTORIUS – the thigh muscle which is extended when sitting cross-legged, as a tailor.
sartor		See sarcio.
sarx; sarcos	G	Flesh, muscles; of these. SARCOMA – a tumour arising from muscle, bone, cartilage or connective tissue.
satyros	G	A satyr, lewd man. SATYRIASIS – excessive sexual desire in a man.
scala	L	A series of steps, a ladder. SCALA TYMPANI – one of the internal passages of the cochlea.
scalenos	G	Unequal, a triangle with unequal sides. SCALENE MUSCLES – triangular shaped muscles lying between the cervical vertebrae and the ribs.
scaphos	G	A hull, a boat. SCAPHOID – the ankle bone shaped like a boat, *Os naviculare.*
scapula	L	The shoulder blade. SCAPULA.
scatos	G	See scor.
scelos	G	The (whole) leg. SCELALGIA – pain in the leg.
schesis	G	Permanent state; retention. SIALOSCHESIS – retention of salivary secretion.
schisis	G	Cleavage, split. SCHISTOSOMA – a trematode parasite in which the female has a cleft along the length of the body.
schizo	G	To split (longitudinally). SCHIZOPROSOPIA – fissure of the face, such as hare-lip, cleft-palate, etc.
sciros	G	A hard covering, of land, cement or skin. SCIRUS –

		a hard outer layer in certain integumentary cancers. Sometimes improperly scirrhus.
scirrhos		See **sciros**.
scleros	G	Hard. SCLEROSIS – hardening by induration, often after inflammation in the nervous and circulatory systems.
scolex	G	A worm, grub. SCOLEX – the "head" of a tapeworm bearing attachment suckers and hooks.
scolios	G	Twisted, crooked, bent sideways. SCOLIOSIS – a lateral bend in the spine.
scopeo	G	To look at something. MICROSCOPE.
scor; scatos	G	Dung, ordure; of these. SCATOLOGY – the study of faeces.
scorbutus	L	Scurvy. SCORBUTIC – pertaining to scurvy.
scotos	G	Darkness, blindness. SCOTOMA – a part of the visual field with reduced visual sensitivity.
scrofa	L	A sow, originally thought to suffer from the disease: SCROFULA – a tubercular disease of the lymph nodes.
scybalon	G	Refuse, excrement. SCYBALA – dry hard faeces in the gut.
sebum	L	Grease. SEBORRHOEA – excessive secretion of sebum and the dermatitis this causes.
seco; sectum	L	To cut, sever; divided. DISSECTION – subdivision of a structure, often a dead animal.
seio	G	To shake, quake, agitate. ODONTOSEISIS – having loose teeth.
selene	G	The moon, the lunar month. SELENODONT – having teeth on which there are crescentic ridges.
sella	L	A seat, stool. SELLA TURCICA – a depression in the sphenoid bone, shaped like a Turkish saddle, which accommodates the pituitary gland.
semeion	G	A sign, symptom. SEMEIOTICS – the study of disease signs and symptoms.
semen	L	Seed of plants or animals. SEMINAL – relating to semen.
semis	L	Half. SEMI-flexion – a position midway between flexion and extension.

sentio; sensum	L	To feel, perceive; felt. SENSORY.
sepsis	G	Putrefaction, fermentation, decay. SEPSIS.
septum		See **saeptum.**
sequestrum	L	Something placed apart to be preserved, a deposit. SEQUESTRUM – a dead piece of bone which separates from a healthy bone.
sero		See **serum.**
serpo	L	To creep, crawl. SERPIGINOUS – of skin lesions which spread out rather irregularly, e.g., ringworm. See also **herpo.**
serratus	L	Saw-toothed. SERRATION.
serum	L	Whey, watery exudate. SEROLIPASE – lipase found in blood serum.
sesame	G	Sesame, its seeds, shaped so. SESAMOID – of a small piece of bone often embedded in a tendon or synovial capsule.
seta		See **saeta.**
siagon	G	The jaw-bone. SIAGONAGRA – maxillary pain.
sialon	G	Saliva, synovial fluid. SIALADENITIS – inflammation of the salivary gland.
siccus	L	Dry. SICCUS.
sideros	G	Iron. SIDEROSIS – excess of iron in the body.
sigma	G,L	S- or C-shaped, crescentic. In Latin, used to mean semi-circular. SIGMOID (COLON).
silex	G	Flint, silica. SILICOSIS – pneumoconiosis from inhalation of stone particles containing silica.
sinciput	L	Half a head (semi-caput); the brain. SINCIPUT – the anterior and upper part of the head.
sinus	L	A curve, bay, hollow. SINUSITIS – inflammation of the sinuses.
sis		See **iasis.**
sitos	G	Food, grain, bread, fodder. SITOMANIA – abnormal craving for food.
skato		See **scor.**
skeletos	G	A dried-up body, mummy, skeleton. SKELETON.
skepto	G	To lean on, simulate, pretend. SKEPTOPHYLAXIS – a desensitization acquired by injecting one or several small doses of the provoking factor.

skia	G	A shadow, shade. SKIAGRAM – an X-ray picture.
smemma, smegma	G	Soap, unguent, detergent. SMEGMA – preputial, sebaceous secretion.
solea	L	The leather sole piece of a sandal; so shaped. SOLEUS – a muscle of the lower leg.
solen	G	A channel, pipe. DACRYOSOLENITIS – inflammation of the lacrimal duct.
soma; somatos	G	The body; of it. SOMATIC.
somnus	L	Sleep. SOMNAMBULIST – one who walks in his or her sleep.
sonor, sonus	L	Sound, noise. SONOMETER – an instrument used for measuring acuteness of hearing.
sopor	L	Deep sleep, lethargy. SOPORIFIC – inducing deep sleep.
spadon	G	A tear, spasm. HYPOSPADIA – having the male urethral opening on the underside of the penis or on the perineum.
span(i)os	G	Rare, scarce; seldom. SPANOPNOEA – slow, deep breathing.
spao	G	To tear apart, draw out. To cause convulsions or spasms. See spasmos and spadon.
spasmos	G	Convulsion, spasm. SPASMOLYTIC – abating or abolishing spasms. See spao.
spastic		See spao and spasmos.
spectrum	L	An image or apparition. SPECTROGRAM – a record of vibrations arranged according to their constituent wavelengths.
speculum	L	A mirror. SPECULUM – a device for obtaining a view of the interior of a cavity or passage.
speira	G	Twisted, wound together. SPIROCHAETE – a spirally-formed bacterium.
sperma; spermatikos	G	Seed, semen; seminal. SPERM – the male gamete.
sphacelos	G	Gangrene, caries, spasm. SPHACELATE – to become necrotic, gangrenous or mortified.
sphen	G	A wedge, shaped so. SPHENOID.
sphincter	G	A tight band, a muscle closing an opening. SPHINCTER – an annular muscle around a passage or opening.

sphingo	G	To bind tightly, tie. SPHINGOLIPID – a particular group of lipids found in the brain and in nervous tissue.
sphygmos	G	The pulse, the beating of the heart. SPHYGMOMANOMETER – an instrument for measuring arterial blood pressure.
sphyra	G	A hammer, mallet. SPHYRECTOMY – removal of the malleus bone.
sphyxis		See **sphygmos.**
spira		See **speira.**
splanchnon	G	An internal organ, one of the viscera. SPLANCHNIC – pertaining to the viscera.
splen	G	The spleen. SPLENITIS – inflammation of the spleen.
spodos	G	Ashes, dust, lava. SPODOGENOUS – producing waste materials.
spondylos	G	A vertebra. SPONDYLOSIS – osteoarthritic degeneration, especially of the vertebral joints.
squama	L	A scale of fish or armour, i.e., plate like. SQUAMOUS.
stabilis	L	Stable, reliable. THERMOSTABLE – not much affected by external temperature changes.
stal		See **stello.**
stapes	L	A stirrup. STAPES – a bone of this shape in the middle ear.
staphyle	G	1. A bunch of grapes. STAPHYLOCOCCUS – spherical bacteria which accumulate in groups or bundles. 2. The uvula when swollen to resemble a grape. STAPHYLINUS – concerned with the uvula.
stasis	G	Position; the placing or condition of something. BACTERIOSTATIC – preventing further multiplication in a bacterial population.
statos	G	Placed, standing. PROSTATE – the gland at the base of the penis which contributes to seminal fluid.
staxis	G	Dripping (of blood). EPISTAXIS – nose-bleeding.
stear; steatos	G	Tallow, fat, suet; of these. STEATORRHOEA – excessive unabsorbed fat in the faeces.

stella, stellula	L	A star, a little star. STELLATE – a star or rosette-shaped structure, e.g., the stellate ganglion.
stello	G	To start, make ready, make costive. PERISTALSIS – travelling waves of contraction, moving the contents of tubular organs.
stenos	G	Narrow, meagre. STENOSIS – a narrowed passage, duct or tube.
stephanos	G	An encircling structure. STEPHANION – the point of intersection of the superior temporal and coronal planes on the side of the skull.
stercus	L	Dung, excrement. STERCORACEOUS – containing faeces.
stereo	G	To be deprived, to be robbed of something. HALISTERESIS – demineralization of the bones, osteomalacia.
stereos	G	Solid, hard, firm, of three dimensions. ASTEREOGNOSIS – tactile amnesia, inability to recognize objects by touch.
sternon	G	The chest, breast. STERNAL – pertaining to the chest.
stethos	G	The breast, chest. STETHOSCOPE – an instrument for listening to body sounds.
sthenos	G	Strength, power. ASTHENIA – weakness, lack of strength.
stichos	G	A file, row of men, a line of verse. TETRASTICHIASIS – having two rows of eye-lashes on each eyelid.
stigma	G	A tattoo, mark, spot. ASTIGMATISM – faulty refraction in the eye, giving an image which is not focussed to a point.
stole		See **stello**; see also **diastole** and **systole**.
stoma; **stomatos**	G	The mouth; oral. ANASTOMOSIS – collateral communications amongst blood vessels, spaces or organs.
stomachos	G	The throat, gullet; stomach. STOMACH.
strabismos	G	Squinting. STRABISMUS – squinting, having the axes of vision in the eyes not coincident.
streptos	G	Easily twisted, pliant, twisted; linked metal in

chain-mail. STREPTOCOCCUS – bacteria which occur in pairs or chains.

stria	L	A furrow. STRIAE – fine lines, bands or streaks.
strict		See **stringo.**
strideo	L	To grate, hiss, screech. STRIDEO – a harsh sound in certain respiratory dysfunctions.
stringo; **strictum**	L	To bind, draw together, pluck; bound. CONSTRICTION.
stroma	G	Something spread out to sit or lie on. Now, the supporting matrix of an organ, not the parenchyma. STROMA.
strongylos	G	Round, spherical, compact. STRONGYLOSIS – infection with the parasitic nematode worm, *Strongylus.*
stroph		See **streptos.**
stropheus	G	A door hinge or pivot; a vertebra. STROPHEUS – the axis vertebra.
struma	L	A scrofulous tumour, a goitre. STRUMA.
stylos	G	A column, pillar. STYLOID – shaped like a pillar.
stypteria	G	Alum, astringent earth. STYPTIC – an astringent substance used to hinder bleeding.
sub	L	Under, beneath, close to. SUBLINGUAL – under the tongue.
subsulto	L	To leap. SUBSULTUS – spasmodic movements, especially those seen in typhoid.
subtilis	L	Fine, slender. BACILLUS SUBTILIS.
succedaneus	L	Taking another's place. SUCCEDANEUM – a substitute, e.g., a drug used in place of another.
succenturio	L	To substitute. SUCCENTURIATE – accessory, acting as a substitute.
suc(c)us	L	A juice, or sap. SUCCUS ENTERICUS – the secretion of the glands of the ileum wall.
sudor	L	Sweat. SUDORIFIC – something causing sweating.
suf		See **sub.**
sui	L	One's self. SUICIDE.
sulcus	L	A furrow. SULCUS.
sup		See **sub.**
supinus	L	Bent backwards; lying on the back with the palms upwards. Supinated; (opposite to pronated). SUPINE.

supra	L	Above, over. SUPRAORBITAL – above the orbit.
sura	L	The calf of the leg. SURA.
surditas	L	Deafness. SURDITAS.
sus		See **sub**.
suscipio; **susceptum**	L	To take up; taken up. INTUSSUSCEPTION – a process of protoplasmic growth by absorption of material at a molecular or microscopical level, not by apposition. Also prolapse of one part of the intestine longitudinally into an adjacent part.
sy		See **syn**.
sycon	G	A fig, shaped so; a large wart on the eyelid; similar tumours or warts. SYCOSIS – ulceration of hair follicles.
syl		See **syn**.
sym		See **syn**.
symptoma	G	A chance, accident, property, symptom. SYMPTOM – an indication of disease or dysfunction noticeable by the patient.
syn	G	United, together with. SYNGAMY – the fusion of two gametes.
synecho	G	To hold together. SYNECHIA – abnormal adhesions, such as that of the iris to the cornea or lens.
synovialis	L	A nutritive fluid especially of the joints. The origin of this word is uncertain. SYNOVIAL.
syrinx	G	A cylindrical pipe or structure. SYRINGOMYELIA – a condition of having liquid-filled vesicles in the spinal cord.
systole	G	A contraction. SYSTOLE.
syzygia	G	Close union, a pair; yoked together. SYZYGY – the contiguous fusion of two organisms, but without loss of identity; the suture or fusion of a joint.

T

tabes	L	Wasting away. TABES DORSALIS – a late syphilitic degeneration of the nerves of the dorsal columns of the spinal cord, causing numerous and various symptoms.

tachys	G	Fast, rapid. TACHYCARDIA – abnormally high heart rate.
tact		See **tango** or **tasso**.
tagma	G	An ordinance, arrangement. NEUROTAGMA – linear pattern of the structure of a nerve cell. See also **tasso, taxis**.
tainia	G	A band, ribbon; tapeworm. TAENIA COLI – a longitudinal strip of muscle on the colon.
talus	L	The ankle, the astragulus bone. TALIPES – clubfoot.
tango; tactum	L	To touch; touched. TACTILE.
tapes, tapetion	G	A carpet, bedspread. TAPETUM – a covering structure or membrane.
tarasso	G	To trouble the mind, agitate, disorder. ATARAXY – perfect peace of mind.
taraxy		See **tarasso**.
tardus	L	Slow, tardy. TARDIVE – of a disease whose characteristics develop late, or after a delay.
tar	G	See **tarasso**.
tarsos	G	1. Basket-work; a flat reed mat; the sole of the foot; the ankle. TARSUS – the ankle joint. 2. The rim of the eyelid with the eye-lashes. TARSORRHAPHY – suturing the eyelids together, wholly or partly.
tasso	G	To place in order. ATACTIC – disorderly. See also **tagma**.
taxis	G	An arrangement, order. ATAXIA – absence or disturbance of muscular coordination. See also **tagma, tasso**.
tectum	L	A roof, covering. TECTUM – the dorsum of the mesencephalon.
tego	L	To cover. INTEGUMENT – external covering of the body.
teichos	G	A wall, circumferential fortification. TEICHOPSIA – the illusion of seeing a flickering zig-zag or wall-like line of light, sometimes associated with migraine.
teinesmos	G	A straining, vain attempt to defaecate or urinate. TENESMUS.

teino	G	To stretch, strain, extend. OPISTHOTONOS – severe bending of the body so the back is concave. See also **tonos, tetanos** and **tendo.**
tela	L	A web, something woven. TELAE – web-like membranes.
tele	G	Far away, at a distance. TELEMETRY – recording and measuring at a distance by means of radio signals.
telos	G	The end, culmination; the highest authority. TELENCEPHALON – the embryonic precursor from which arise the cerebral hemispheres.
temno	G	To cut, sever. CORDOTOMY – dividing the spinal cord.
tempus	L	The temples (of the head). TEMPORAL – pertaining to the lateral region of the head, superior to the zygomatic arch.
tenacula	L	Forceps. TENACULUM – something which holds e.g., a hook-shaped instrument; or a band of fibrous tissue within the body.
tendo; tensum	L	To extend; stretched. EXTENSOR – a muscle extending a limb.
tene		See **tainia.**
tenon	G	A sinew, tendon. TENDON.
tensio		See **tendo.**
tentorium	L	A tent, shaped so. TENTORIUM.
teras	G	A marvel, monster, omen. TERATOLOGY – the study of congenital malformations.
teres; teretis	L	Round; smoothed. TERES – long, and round in cross-section, e.g., like a limb muscle.
tergum	L	The back, behind. VIS-A-TERGO – the residual pressure in the veins after the blood has passed through the arterioles and capillaries.
tero; tritum	L	To rub, wear away; rubbed. INTERTRIGO – chafing of the skin.
tetanos	G	Stretched, taut, strained. TETANUS – muscle contraction producing maintained tension. See **teino.**
tetra	G	Four (used only as a prefix). TETRAPLEGIA – paralysis of all four limbs.

thalame	G	A hidden lair; used of the cavities of the body, the ventricles of the heart, the sinuses of cranial bones. THALAMUS – a part of the diencephalon adjacent to the third ventricle.
thalassa	G	The sea, especially the Mediterranean. THALASSAEMIA – a disease of haemoglobin production. The name derives from the Mediterranean Sea, where it was first investigated.
thanatos	G	Death. EUTHANASIA – an easy and painless death, and methods to promote this.
theca	G	A case, chest, tomb. THECA – an enclosing sheath or sheet of tissue.
theion	G	Brimstone, sulphur. THIOGENIC – synthesizing more complex sulphur compounds from hydrogen sulphide.
thele	G	A teat, nipple. THELITIS – inflammation of the nipple.
thelium		A membrane. EPITHELIUM. Thelium is a late invention and not found in Latin or Greek.
thelys	G	Female, tender, delicate, soft. EPITHELIUM – the internal or external covering layer of a structure.
thema		See **thesis**.
thenar	G	The palm of the hand. THENAR.
therapeuo	G	To care for medically. THERAPEUTICS.
therme	G	Heat. HYPOTHERMIA – having an abnormally low body temperature.
thesis	G	A setting, arranging, placing. SYNTHESIS – putting things together, opposite to analysis.
thlao	G	To crush, bruise. ENTHLASIS – skull fracture with depression of the bony fragments.
thlibo; thlipsis	G	To press, squeeze, chafe; pressure. ONCOTHLIPSIS – pressure from the growth of the tumour.
threpteos	G	To be nourished. THREPSOLOGY – the study of nutrition.
thrix; trichos	G	A hair; hairy. TRICHIASIS – ingrowing hairs.
thrombos	G	A lump, clot. THROMBOSIS – the formation or presence of a thrombus.
thymos	G	The soul, mind, spirit. Also the heart, supposedly

the seat of the emotions. (a) CYCLOTHYMIA – exaggerated cyclic changes of mood from elation to depresssion. (b) THYMUS – a diffuse gland partly covering the heart and great vessels. Cf. **phren** and **psyche.**

thyreoeides G An oblong shield; the thyroid cartilage which has this shape. THYROID – the laryngeal cartilage and the gland adjacent to it.

tillo G To pluck or pull out, hair, feathers, leaves. ONYCHOTILLOMANIA – an obsessional picking at the nails.

tinea L A gnawing worm, larva of a moth. TINEA – various fungal skin diseases; ringworm.

tinnitus L Ringing, tinkling, jangling noise. TINNITUS – crackling, ringing or other noises arising within the ears, but also sometimes delusive.

titheme G A nurse. DYSTITHIA – difficulty in suckling.

tmesis G Cutting, ravaging. NEUROTMESIS – severance or partial severance of a nerve preventing recovery of function. See **temno.** Cf. neurapraxia.

tocos G Offspring, birth. DYSTOCIA – difficulty in parturition.

tofus L Porous stone, tufa. TOFUS – synovial deposition of calcereous material, urates, etc., in gout.

tomus G Sharp, cutting. Also a slice, piece. See **temno.**

ton, tone   See **tonos.**

tonos G The tension in something, especially a string or cord and the sound this can give. TONUS – the resting tension in muscles. See **teino.**

tophus   See **tofus.**

topos G A place, position. ECTOPIC – of something displaced, in an anomalous position.

tormina L Colic. TORMINA.

tortum L Crooked, twisted. TORTICOLLIS – wry or twisted neck.

torus, torulus L A swelling, protuberance. TORUS.

toxon G A bow, and later transferred to the poison in which arrows were dipped. TOXIC – poisonous.

trabecula	L	A little beam, bar. TRABECULAE – strands of tissue which maintain something in position. Cf. **tenaculum**
trachelos	G	The neck and throat. TRACHELOCYLLOSIS – wryneck, torticollis.
trachys	G	Rough, rugged, hard. (Possibly mistaking the trachea for a coarse artery.) TRACHEA – the windpipe. Cf. **bronchus**
tract		See **traho.**
tragos	G	The male goat, the age of puberty, lewdness. TRAGUS – the projection of the pinna on which a tuft of hairs grows (supposed to resemble the beard of a goat).
traho; tractus	L	To draw or pull along; drawn along. PROTRACTOR – an instrument for removing foreign bodies from wounds; a muscle serving to pull forward or extend a limb.
trans	L	Beyond, to the other side. TRANSFUSION.
trauma	G	A wound, damage, hurt. TRAUMATIC – concerned with an inflicted injury.
trepanon		See **trypanon.**
trephine, trefin	?	TREPHINE – a small trepan, an instrument for cutting out a disc from a structure. See **trypanon.** The origin of this word is uncertain.
trepho	G	To cause to grow, foster. TREPHOCYTE – a cell which nourishes other cells.
trepo	G	To turn. TREPONEMA – spirally formed, often parasitic, bacteria.
tresis	G	A perforationn or orifice. ATRESIA – a congenital absence of a normal opening.
tretos	G	Perforated. See **tresis.**
trias	G	Three. TRIAD – a collection of three. See also **ad.**
tribo	G	To rub, wear out, pound, lay waste. ENTRIPSIS – rubbing ointment on the skin.
trich, trix		See **thrix.**
trigeminus	L	Triplets, threefold. TRIGEMINUS – the fifth cranial nerve which has three major branches.
trigo		See **tero.**

trimester	L	A period of 3 months (12 weeks). TRIMESTER – a period of three months, especially in pregnancy.
triphthesomai	G	To be wasted. TRIPHTHAEMIA – retention of waste products in the blood. From **tribo.**
tripsis		See **tribo.**
trismos	G	Grating, grinding. TRISMUS – spasm of the masticatory muscles, an early symptom of tetanus.
tritura	L	The threshing of corn. TRITURATION – the grinding of food or drugs.
trocar, trochar	F	'Trois carré', i.e., having three sides. TROCAR – an instrument used for introduing a catheter into the body.
trochos	G	A wheel, shaped so. TROCHLEA – one of several structures in the body, functioning or shaped as a pulley.
tromos	G	A trembling, quaking, quivering. TROMOMANIA – delirium tremens.
trop		See **trepo** and **tropos.**
trophe	G	Nourishment, food. TROPHOBLAST – a cell on the outer surface of the embryo which takes up nutrients from the endometrium.
tropos	G	A way or direction to be followed; a habit, custom. NEUROTROPIC – affecting the nervous system.
trosis	G	An injury. NEUROTROSIS – neurotrauma.
trudo; trusum	L	To push, press; pushed. DETRUSOR – the muscle of the bladder wall which expels the urine.
trypanon	G	An auger, boring tool. TREPANNING – an old type of trephining.
trypao	G	To pierce through. CEPHALOTRYPESIS – trephining of the cranium.
tuber, tuberculum	L	A hump, a little swelling. TUBERCULAR.
tumeo; tumesco	L	To be swollen; to begin to swell. TUMOUR – a swelling.
tunica	L	An (under) garment for either men or women. TUNICA – membranous organ sheath.
turbo; turbinis	L	A whirlwind, a spinnning top, rotation; of these. TURBINATE – scroll-shaped nasal bones.

tussi	L	A cough. TUSSIS.
tylos	G	A knob, callus. OSTEOTYLUS – callus forming of the end of a broken bone.
tympanon	G	A drum. TYMPANIC MEMBRANE – the ear drum.
typhlon	G	Pertaining to the caecum. TYPHLITIS – inflammation of the caecum.
typhlos	G	Blind. TYPHLOLOGY – information and knowledge about blindness.
typhos	G	A fever accompanied by stupor. TYPHOID – like typhus, a disease with stupor, delirium and fever.
typos	G	A blow, struck image, type. ZELOTYPIA – morbid zeal or jealousy.
tyros	G	Cheese. TYROTOXIN – a poison sometimes found in dairy produce.

U

ul, ula, ule, ulo		See **oule** or **oulon**.
ulcus	L	A sore, ulcer, excrescence. ULCER.
ulna	L	The elbow, arm. ULNA – the fore-arm bone forming the elbow.
ultra	L	Beyond. ULTRASONIC – applied to sound with a frequency greater than about 20 kHz.
umbilicus	L	The navel, centre of a roll or whorl. UMBILICUS – the scar marking the site of the foetal connection to the umbilical cord.
umbo	L	The central boss of a shield, a prominence. UMBONATE – having the form of a boss or knob.
uncus	L	A hook. UNCINATE – hook-shaped.
unguentum	L	Ointment, salve, perfume. UNGUENTUM.
unguis	L	A nail, claw. SUBUNGUAL – beneath the nail. Cf. **onyx**.
unus, uni	L	One. UNILATERAL – on one side only.
ur		See **ouron**.
urachos		See **ourachos**.
uraniscos		See **ouranos**.

urceus	L	An earthenware pitcher, large jug. URCEOLOATE – shaped like a jug.
uresis		See **oureo.**
urtica	L	A stinging-nettle. URTICARIA – a skin reaction, usually temporary, with wheals and itching.
utriculus	L	A small sac. UTRICLE.
uva	L	A bunch of grapes. UVEITIS – inflammation of the iris, ciliary body and the choroid layer of the eye.
uvula	L	A little grape, shaped so. UVULA – a small fleshy structure, especially that of the soft palate.

V

vacca	L	A cow. VACCINIA – cowpox.
vacuus	L	Empty, void. VACUOLE – a cavity in protoplasm.
vagina	L	A scabbard, sheath. VAGINA – a sheathlike structure particularly applied to the canal between the vulva and the uterus.
vagus	L	Wandering. VAGUS – the tenth cranial nerve, innervating many viscera.
valgus	L	Bow-legged. Now, bent outwards, away from the mid-line. TALIPES VALGUS – a condition in which the heel is rotated outwards.
vallate		See **vallum.**
vallecula	L	A little valley, hollow. VALLECULA – a small anatomical depression or hollow.
vallum	L	A wall, stockade, palisade. VALLUM – the fold of skin covering the sides and base of a nail.
varius	L	Diverse, variegated. VARIOLOID – a mild form, or attack, of smallpox.
varix, varices	L	Varicose vein(s). VARICOSE.
varus	L	Knock-kneed. Now, bent in towards the midline. TALIPES VARUS – a condition in which the heel is rotated inwards.
vas	L	A vessel. VAS DEFERENS – the duct conveying semen from the epididymis to the urethra in males.
vasculum	L	A small vessel. VASCULAR.

vector		See **veho**.
vegetus	L	Lively, vigorous. VEGETAL – concerned with growth and nutrition, and also the involuntary functions of the body.
veho; vectum	L	To carry, convey; carried. VECTOR – an organism acting as a carrier of a disease organism.
vello; vulsum	L	To pull, twitch; pulled. CONVULSION – strong involuntary contractions of skeletal muscles.
velum	L	A curtain, covering. VELUM – a membrane covering another part.
vena	L	A vein. VENESECTION – cutting open a vein.
veneno	L	To poison. VENENATION – poisoning.
venereus	L	Appertaining to Venus, goddess of love. VENEREAL – depending on sexual contact.
venter	L	The belly, lower abdomen. VENTRAL – the under-surface of a animal or part of an animal.
vermis	L	A worm. VERMIFORM – wormlike.
vernix	L	Varnish. VERNIX CASEOSA – a fatty, cheesy deposit on the skin of a foetus.
verruca	L	A wart, excrescence. VERRUCAE – warts of viral origin and similar excrescences.
versus	L	Towards, in the direction of. RETROVERSION – the rotation of an organ backwards.
vertex	L	A whirlpool, whorl; the crown of the head. VERTEX – the summit of something, especially the cranium.
vertigo	L	A turning, revolution. VERTIGO – a sensation of rotation either subjective or objective.
vesica	L	A bladder. VESICOENTERIC – concerned with the bladder and gut.
vesicula	L	A small bladder. VESICULAR – pertaining to small bladders or sacs.
vestibulum	L	An entrance, court-yard. VESTIBULE – the entrance region of a tube or passage.
vestigium	L	A footprint, track, mark, spoor. VESTIGIUM – a nonfunctional remnant or relic in the adult, particularly of structures which were functional in the embryo and foetus.

vestis	L	A garment, covering. TRANSVESTISM – dressing as one of the opposite sex, or the desire to do so.
vibro	L	To shake, make vibrate, tremble. VIBRIO – a genus of microorganisms which are actively motile.
villus	L	A tuft of shaggy hair. VILLUS – a fine projection on the wall of the gut.
vinculum	L	A fetter, chain, bond. VINCULUM – a band, or similar structure.
vir; virilis	L	A man; masculine. VIRILISM – the development of male characteristics in the female.
virus	L	Slime, poison. VIROLOGY – study of virus diseases and viruses.
vis; vires	L	Force(s), power(s), strength(s). VIS-A-TERGO – the residual pressure in the veins after the blood has passed through the arterioles and capillaries.
viscum	L	Mistletoe, bird lime, i.e., a sticky substance. VISCID.
viscus, viscera	L	Internal organ(s). VISCERA.
vita	L	Life. See **vivus**.
vitreus	L	Made of glass, like glass. VITREODENTINE – a very hard, glass-like dentine.
vivus	L	Alive, living. VIVISECTION – experimentation involving surgical interference on living animals.
vola	L	The hollow of the hand or foot. VOLA.
volo	L	To be willing, to will. VOLITION – the exercise of the power of choosing.
volvo, volutum	L	To turn, twist, revolve. VOLVULUS – obstruction of the gut by twisting.
vomer	L	A plough-share, shaped so. VOMER – the median bone of the nose.
voro	L	To eat greedily, devour. CARNIVORE – a flesh-eating animal.
vortex	L	See **vertex**.
vulnus; vulneris	L	A wound; of this. VULNERATE – to injure.
vulsion		See **vello**.

X

xanthos	G	Yellow, golden in colour. XANTHOCHROMIA – the condition of having a yellow colour, applied to cerebrospinal fluid stained with blood.
xenos	G	A stranger, visitor, guest. AXENIC – applied to a pure culture of microorganisms, or a germ-free animal.
xeo	G	To scrape, whittle. APOXESIS – removal of debris from a tooth socket.
xeros	G	Dry. XERODERM – dry skin, a mild type of ichthyosis.
xesis		See **xeo**.
xiphos	G	A sword, shaped so. XIPHOID.
xysma	G	Scrapings. XYSMA – fragments, especially of cell membranes in diarrhoeic faeces.
xyster	G	An engraving tool, scraper, rasp, file. XYSTER – a surgical file or rasp.

Z

zelos	G	Jealousy, zeal, fervour. ZELOTYPIA – morbid zeal or jealousy.
zemia	G	Loss, penalty. SIALOZEMIA – involuntary secretion of saliva.
zestos	G	Hot, boiling. ZESTOCAUTERY – a cautery using superheated steam.
zone, zonula	L	A girdle, belt. ZONULA CILIARIS – a girdle of fibres holding the lens of the eye in place.
zoon	G	Animal, living thing. SPERMATOZOON – the male gamete.
zoster	G	A warrior's belt; a girdle. ZOSTRIFORM – like herpes zoster.
zygon	G	A yoke, pair, connecting beam. ZYGOMA – a bone of the face, the zygomatic bone.
zyme	G	Leaven, yeast. ENZYME – a proteinaceous catalyst, a ferment.

Section 2

Medical terms divided into their constituent parts

A list of medical words subdivided to show the roots from which they are formed. Each root word is given in Section 1, although sometimes the spelling of the root word, as used today in English, varies from the original classical form.

Languages are the pedigree of nations.

Samuel Johnson

A

a basia
ab duct
ab epithymia
aborti facient
a boulia
a campsia
acantho kerato dermia
acar iasis
a cathexia
a cathisia
a cephalous
aces odyne
aceton aemia
a chalasia
a chlor hydria
a chlor opsia
a cholia
a chondro plasia
a chrestic
a chromat opsia
a chylia
a cleisto cardia
acm aesthesia
acon uresis
a coria
acos gnosis
a cratia
a crat uresis
acro dolicho melia
acro dynia
acro megaly
acr omion
acro phobia
actino mycetes
acu puncture
acus tenaculum

a cyan osis
a cyesis
adamanto blast
ad duct
adelo morphic
aden ectomy
aden oid
aden oma
adeno pathy
adeno scler osis
a dia docho kinesia
a dia phoresis
ad renal
aego broncho phony
aer odont algia
aero urethro scope
aer piezo therapy
aesthesio genic
aetio logy
a geusia
a glossia
a gnosia
a gomph osis
agora phobia
a graphia
ailuro philia
ailuro phobia
a knepha scopia
alae nasi
aleo cyte
a lexia
alexo cyte
algo meter
allach aesthesia
allant iasis
allanto angio pagous
allanto genesis
allelo morph

allelo taxia
all ergic
allo aesthesia
allo cortex
allo graft
allotrio guestia
allotrio phagy
allo ploid
alveolo clasis
amaur osis
ambly opia
ambo ceptor
amel genesis
amelo genesis
a metr opia
amnesia
amnio centesis
amoeb oid
amphi arkyo chrome
amphi coelus
ampho philic
amyl oid osis
amylos uria
amyl uria
a myo trophy
ana bolism
ana clasis
ana clitic
an acousis
ana dipsia
an aemia
an aesthesia
an akousis
ana lepsis
an algesia
ana mnesis
ana phylaxis
an arthria

ana stom osis
ancon ad
ancylo stoma
andro gen
andro gyne
an eurysm
angi itis
angio gram
angi oma
angio psathyr osis
angio sarc oma
angio tripsy
an hidr osis
an hydrous
an icteric
an iridia
an iso coria
an iso melia
an iso metr opia
ankylo blepharon
ankylo glossia
ankyl osis
ankylo stoma
an odyne
a nomia
an orchis
an orexia
an osmia
ant agonist
ante flexion
ante grade
ante natal
antero grade
anthropo logy
anti biotic
anti dote
anti posia
anti septic

antro scope
a phasia
aphe phobia
a phthongia
apico lysis
a pnoea
apo neur osis
apo physis
apo xesis
appendic itis
a pselaphesia
a pyretic
arachno dactylia
arachn oid
arch enteron
argyro phil
aristo genic
arkyo chrome
arrheno blast oma
arrheno genic
arterio scler osis
arthr itis
arthro cleisis
arthro desis
arthro gryphosis
arthro kleisis
arthro plasty
arthr osis
aryten oid
ascar iasis
a spermia
a sphyxia
a stereo gnosis
a sthenic
a stigmatism
astro cyt oma
a syn desis
a tactic

a tar algesia
a taraxia
a taxia
atel ectasis
ather oma
ather osis
a threpsia
a tresia
a treto stomia
a trichous
a trophic
a trophy
audio metry
auri nasal
aut arcesis
auto chthon
auto immune
auto nomic
a xenic
axio labial
a zygous

B

bacterio stasis
balan itis
balano blenno rrhoea
balano chlamyd itis
balano coel
balano posth itis
balneo therapy
basi hy oid
basi petal
basi phil
bathmo tropic
batho morphic
bathy an aesthesia
bathy cardia

bathy pnoea
bi ceps
bi cornuate
bi cuspid
bi fid
bi furcate
bili rubin
bio logy
bi penni form
blasto cyst
blasto myc osis
blenno rrhoea
blephar aden itis
blepharo chalasis
blepharo ptosis
blepharo synechia
brachy cephalic
brachy gnathous
brady cardia
brady lalia
bromato logy
brom hidr osis
broncho scope
bruxo mania
bubon algia
bubono coel
bu limy
bun odont
buno selen odont
burs itis
byssin osis

C

cac hexia
caco genesis
caco geusia
caco melia

cac osmia
caeno genesis
calci pexy
calci phylaxis
cali sthenics
campto cormia
campto dactyly
campto spasm
candid aemia
candid iasis
cantho plasty
cantho rrhaphy
cantho tomy
carbo hydrate
carcin oma
cardi ectasis
cardio gram
cardio megaly
cardio myo lip osis
cardio myo pexy
cardio necr osis
cardio sphygmo graph
carni fication
carni vore
carpo meta
carpal
carpo ptosis
caseino gen
caseo genous
caseo serum
cata bolism
cata clonus
cata lepsy
cata lyst
cata phoresis
cata phrenia
cata tropia
caud ad

caus algia
cen aesthesia
centri fugal
cephal algia
cephalo coel
cephalo trypesis
Cerco monas
cerco pithec oid
cerebro mening itis
cerebro spinal
cerebro vascular
cero lysin
cheil itis
cheilo gnatho schisis
chiro podist
chol angio gram
chol ascos
chol agogue
chole bili rubin
chole cyst endysis
chole cysto kinin
chole docho lith iasis
chole dochus
chol emesis
chole poiesis
chole steat oma
cholin ergic
chondro cranium
chondro sarc oma
chord itis
chordo tomy
chor oid eremia
chromato phil
chromato lysis
chromo crinia
chromo paric
chromo pexis
chromo phil

chromo some
chron axie
chrono gnosis
croto plast
chryso derma
chryso iasis
chryso phoresis
chryso therapy
cingul ectomy
cingulumo tomy
cion itis
ciono rrhaphy
circa dian
circum vallate
cirs ectomy
cirs en chysis
cirso cele
cirs omphalos
cyt oma
clasmat osis
clasto thrix
claustro phobia
cleid agra
cleid arthr itis
cleido costal
cleido mast oid
cleido rrhexis
cleido tripsy
clino meter
cnemo scoli osis
coccygeo dynia
cochle itis
coel onychia
col ectomy
coleo cyst itis
colla gen
coll oid
coll oid clasia

coll oid phagia
col lutory
colo stomy
colp itis
colpo centesis
colpo cleisis
colp odynia
colpo episio rrhaphy
colpo sten osis
con ception
conchi form
concho scope
conio fibr osis
conio lymph stasis
conio toxic osis
con jugate
con junctiva
con strict
contra ceptive
con vulsion
copi opia
copro lalia
copro phagia
copro phobia
copro porphyrin
copro stasis
cordo tomy
coron oid
cotyl oid
cox algia
cranio facial
cranio syn ost osis
cranio tabes
cranio trypesis
creno therapy
cribri form
cric oid
crymo an aesthesia

crymo therapy
cryo cardio plegia
cryo crit
cryo genic
cryo phylactic
cryo stat
cryo surgery
crypto mnesia
crypt orchidism
cunei form
cyan haemo globin
cyan osis
cyclo thymia
cyno cephalic
cyn odont
cyn orexia
cyo genic
cyo phoric
cyst itis
cysto elytro plasty
cysto lith iasis
cyto penia
cyto toxic

D

dacry agog a tresia
dacryo aden ectomy
dacryo cyst ectomy
dacryo cysto rhino stomy
dacryo helc osis
dacryo solen itis
dactylo camps odynia
dactylo gryph osis
dactylo megaly
de cidua
de faecate
de furfuration

de glutition
delt oid
de mentia
de mulcent
dent agra
dento alveolar
deonto logy
de pilate
der encephalo coel
dermato dys plasia
dermato fibr oma
dermato glyphics
dermato phyte
dermato zo iasis
dermato zoon osis
desm oid
desmo logy
desmo pexia
desmo pykn osis
desmo some
de trusor
deuter an opia
dextro cardia
dextro gyration
dia betic
dia crisis
di aeresis
dia gnosis
dia lysis
dia pedesis
dia peiresis
dia rrhoea
dia stasis
di cephalous
dich optic
dich otic
dicho tomy
di chromatic

di coelous
di coria
di gestion
digiti form
dioptro meter
dipl acusis
diplo coccus
diplo karyon
diplo myelia
diplo pagus
dipl opia
di prosopus
dipso mania
dipso phobia
dips osis
di pygus
disco placenta
dis section
di uresis
dolicho cephalic
drepano cyte
duct itis
duodeno chol ange itis
duodeno jejuno stomy
duo parental
dys acusis
dys ana gnosis
dys entery
dys lexia
dys meno rrhoea
dys par eunia

E

eburn itis
ec chym oma
ec chym osis
echino coccus

echino cyte
echin opthalmia
eco logy
ecto derm
ec topic
ect ost osis
ectro genic
ectro melia
ego centric
ego mania
elaio pathy
electro cardio gram
electro encephalo graph
electro myo graphy
eleo meter
eleo plast
eleo pten
em bol phrasia
em bryo
emmetr opia
em peri polesis
em phraxis
em physema
enantio morph
enantio pathic
en capsulate
encephal itis
encephalo coel
encephalo myel itis
endemio logy
endo cardium
endo crin a sthenic
endo gastr itis
endo hernio rrhaphy
endo lysis
endo metri osis
endo metrium
endo phleb itis

end ophthalmus
endo thelio blast oma
end oto scope
endo tox aemia
ensi form
ent amoeb iasis
enter itis
entero cleisis
entero clysis
entero epiplo coel
entero mero coel
entero ptychia
en thlasis
ent iris
ento coel
ento derm
ento zoon
en tripsis
en tropion
en uresis
en zymo logy
eosino phil
ep axial
ependymo blast
ep haptic
ep hebic
epi canthus
epi demic
epi demio logy
epi dermo dys plasia
epi dermo myc osis
epi didymis
epi dural
epi gastrium
e pilation
epi lepsy
epi neural
epi physis

epi physio lysis
epiplo coel
epiplo rrhaphy
episio rrhaphy
episio tomy
epi spadia
epi staxis
epi thelium
epi typhl itis
ep onychium
ep ulis
ep ul osis
erethiso phrenia
erythro cyte
erythro cyto penia
erythro plasia
erythro poiesis
erythr osis
eso cata phora
eso gastr itis
eso tropic
ethm oid
ethno logy
etio logy
eu dia phoresis
eu karyon
eu pepsia
eu phoria
eu pnoeic
eury cephalic
eury somatic
eu thyroid
eu tocia
eu trophic
e version
e vulsion
ex airesis
ex anthem

ex coriation
ex cyt osis
ex eresis
ex foliation
ex halation
exo crine
exo gastr itis
exo genous
exo pathic
ex ost osis
exo thermic
extra dural
extra embryonic
extra placental
extra renal
extra venous

F

falci form
fascio rrhaphy
fibrino genesis
fibrino lysis
fibro cytic
fili form
flavo protein
freno tomy
funicul itis
furuncul osis
fusi form

G

galact agogue
galacto crasia
galacto phlysis
galacto phygous
galacto pyra

gastro algo ken osis
gastro dia tonic
gastro ptosis
gastro staxis
gel osis
gelo therapy
gelo tripsy
genio hy oid
genio plasty
geno cide
geny antr algia
ger iatric
geri odontic
gerio psych osis
geronto logy
gingiv itis
glauc oma
glen oid
gli oma
glio my oma
glomerulo nephr itis
glosso lalia
glosso pyr osis
glosso tilt
glyco gen
glyco genesis
glyco lytic
gnatho dynamo meter
gnatho plasty
gnoto biotic
gnoto phoresis
gonado trophin
gona agra
gon arthr osis
.gone poiesis
gonio scope
gonio tomy
gono campsis

gono coccal
gono rrhoea
gony crotesis
gony ec typ osis
granulo cyte
granulo cyto penia
granul oma
gutturo tetany
gyn andrism
gyn andr oid
gynaeco logy
gynaeco mastia
gyno genesis
gyno pathic
gyr ectomy

H

haem cyto meter
haem angi oma
haema phein
haem arthr osis
haem a sthen osis
haemat hidrosis
haemato chezia
haemato colpo metra
haemat onco metry
haemato salpinx
haemo clastic
haemo dia pedesis
haemo pneuma thorax
haemo poiesis
haemo ptysis
haemo rrhagia
haemo sider osis
haemo stasis
hali steresis
halit osis

halo gen
halo philic
ham arthr itis
hamart oma
hamarto phasia
hapl oid
haplo phase
haplo opia
hapto globin
hapto meter
hebe phrenia
heb oido phrenia
heb osteo tomy
helc osis
helic oid
helico trema
hel oma
helo tomy
hemer al opia
hemi blepsia
hemi an opia
hemi cephalus
hemi glosssal
hemi hyp aesthesia
hemi melia
hepat ectomy
hepatico chole docho stomy
hepato dys trophy
hepato jugular
hepato megaly
hernia plasty
hernia rrhaphy
herp angia
herpeti form
hetero cephalus
hetero chthonous
heter odont
hetero genous

hetero kinesis
hetero meric
hetero nomous
hetero nymous
hetero phthongia
hetero topic
hetero xenous
hetero zyg osis
hidros aden itis
hidr osis
histo clastic
histo cyte
histo lysis
histo teli osis
hodo neuro mere
holo en zyme
holo tonia
holo type
homalo cephalus
homal uria
homeo path
homeo static
homo gamous
homo geneous
homo genous
homo glandular
homoio stasis
homoio therm
homo logous
hom-onomous
homo nymous
homo zygote
hormon poietic
hyal itis
hyalo nyxis
hyalo plasm
hyalo seros itis
hydatid uria

hydati form
hydr agogue
hydr amnion
hydr argyro mania
hydro cenosis
hydro cirso coel
hydro penia
hydro phobia
hydropo therapy
hydro salpinx
hydro ureter
hygieo logy
hygro blepharic
hygr oma
hygro meter
hylo genesis
hylo tropic
hymen ectomy
hymeno tomy
hy oid
hyp acusis
hyp aemia
hyp algesia
hyp ana kinesis
hyper acusis
hyper adip osis
hyper aemia
hyper algia
hyper baric
hyper capnia
hyper chylia
hyper cyt aemia
hyper gonadism
hyper iso tonia
hyper mastic
hyper metr opia
hyper myo trophy
hyper phrenia

hyper placia
hyper pyrexia
hyper tel orism
hyper trich iasis
hyp hedonia
hyphe philia
hypho mycetic
hypno balia
hypo aesthesia
hypo endo crinism
hypo gamma globulin aemia
hypo geusia
hypo kal aemia
hypo myxia
hypo piezia
hypo pnoeic
hypo spadia
hypo sthenia
hypo thymia
hypo vegetative
hyp oxia
hypsi brady cephalic
hypsi conchous
hyps odont
hypso nosus
hyster eurynter
hyster eurysis
hystero cleisis
hyster odynia
hystero laparo tomy
hystero neuro a sthenia
hystero salpingo graphy

I

iamato logy
iath ergy
iatr aliptic

iatro genic
iatro logy
ichor aemia
icho rrhoea
ichthy osis
ideo phrenia
ideo vascular
idio blapsis
idio pathy
idio syn crasy
ileo cysto plasty
ileo procto stomy
ilio psoas
im palpable
impar digitate
im per meable
in cisure
inco stapedial
in durated
in farct
infra costal
infra spinous
infra version
in halation
inio pagus
in nominate
ino blast
ino lith
inos aemia
ino scler osis
ino tropic
in tegument
inter carpal
inter furcal
inter trigo
intra corporeal
intra luminal
intro itus

intro jection
intro version
intus susception
in volucre
ipsi lateral
iri desis
irido coloboma
irido meso dia lysis
irido plegia
irido tomy
ir itis
isch aemia
isch hidr osis
ischio (di)dymia
ischio gyria
ischio melus
ischio rectal
isch uria
is eiconia
iso caloric
iso chronous
iso hydric
iso iconia
ithy kyph osis
ithy lord osis
Ixodes
ixod iasis

J

juxta glomerular
juxt allo cortex
juxta pyloric
juxta spinal

K

kali uresis
kary enchyma

karyo clasis
karyo plasm
karyo theca
keiro spasm
kel ectomy
kel oid
keno phobia
kerat algia
kerat ectasia
kerat ino cyte
kerato helc osis
kerato malacia
kera tome
kerato nyxis
kerato tome
kern icterus
keto genic
keton aemia
keton uria
kinesio logy
kineto graphic
kineto some
kino cilium
kiono tomy
kio tomy
koil onychia
koilo rrhachic
koilo sternia
kraur osis
kyll osis
kymo graph
kypho lordosis
kypho scoli osis
kyph osis

L

labio incisal

labio tenaculum
labio version
lacrimo nasal
lacti ferous
lacti genous
lacto genic
lactos uria
lag ophthalmos
lambd oid
lamelli form
lamin ectomy
lampro phonia
lapar ectomy
laparo colo stomy
laparo toma philia
laparo typhlo tomy
laryng itis
laryngo centesis
laryngo hypo pharynx
laryngo xer osis
latero flexion
latero version
lathyro genic
lecithin aemia
leio my oma
leio trichous
leipo meria
leipo stomia
leipo thymia
lenti conus
lenti form
lepto meninx
lepto mon ad
lepto pella
lepto prosopic
lepto rrhine
leucin osis
leucin uria

leuc onychia
leuco penia
leuco tomy
leuko plakia
leuko virus
lieno gastric
lieno renal
lieno toxic
limo phthisis
limo therapy
lipara cele
lipo dys trophy
lipo hyalin
lip oid osis
lipo meria
lipo stomy
lipo thymia
lipso trichia
lip uria
liss encephalic
lith angio uria
lith ec bole
lith iasis
litho clysmia
litho lapaxy
litho triptic
lochio cyte
lochio stasis
loco motion
logad ectomy
logad itis
log a gnosia
logo clony
logo kophosis
logo rrhoea
logo scope
loph odont
Lopho phora

lopho trichous
lordo scoli osis
lord osis
lox arthron
loxo tomy
luci fugal
luci petal
lumi flavin
lumino phore
lunato malacia
luteo tropin
lyc anthropy
lyco mania
lyc orexia
lymph aden ectomy
lymph angi ectasis
lympho epi theli oma
lyo philic
lyso genic
lyso some
lyso zyme
lysso dexis
lysso phobia

M

macro amylase
macro cheilia
macro cheiria
macr odontia
macro mazia
maculo papular
maculo vesicular
malaco plakia
malleo tomy
mallo chorion
mal occlusion
mamma plasty

mammill itis
mammo gram
mammo graphy
mammo plasty
margino plasty
maschal aden itis
maschal oncus
masso therapy
mast ectomy
mast odynia
mast oid
masto parietal
masto squamous
maxillo palantine
mazo plasia
mecisto cephalic
meconio rrhoea
mecy stasis
medo rrhoea
medullo blast
mega colon
megalo melia
megal opsia
megalo ureter
meion ectic
melan cholia
melano glossia
melan oma
melen emesis
meli cera
melit uria
melo didymus
melon (on)cus
meningo cele
meningo coel
meningo myelo coel
meningo theli oma
meno plania

meno rrhagia
mento anterior
mento labial
mentul agra
mentulo mania
mer algia
mero cox algia
mero gony
mero melia
mes encephalon
mesio gingival
meso appendix
meso cord
meso pneumon
meso rachi schizis
mes ovarium
meta chromasia
meta globulin
meta morph osis
meta plasia
meta stasis
meta syn desis
met haemo globin aemia
metop odynia
metopo pagus
metr algia
metr a tonia
metr ectasis
metr ec topia
metro fibr oma
metro rrhaphy
micro aero philous
micro coccus
micro filar aemia
micro phallus
micro sphygmia
micro thelia
mio cardia

mito chondria
mogi arthria
mogi lalia
mon a thet osis
monili form
mono chroic
mono phyletic
mono plegia
mono syn aptic
mon ovular
mono xenic
morph allaxis
morpho genesis
morph osis
multi gravida
multi locular
muta genesis
my a sthenia
my a tonia
mycet oma
myco derma
myc osis
myco stat
myco toxin
mydr iasis
my ec topia
myel apoplexy
myel itis
myelo cele
myelo meningo coel
myelo plexy
my enteron
myia (ia)sis
myio cephalon
mylo hy oid
myo cele
myo chord itis
myo clonus

myo haemo globin uria
myo kymia
my opia
myo syn izesis
myo ton oid
myringo myc osis
myringo stapedio pexy
myringo tomy
myso philia
myso phobia
myx oedema
myxo poiesis
myxo sarcoma
myxo virus

N

nano cephaly
nano melia
nano soma
narco ana lysis
narco hypnia
narco lepsy
narc osis
naso lacrimal
naso sinus itis
natri uresis
natr uresis
necro mimesis
necr opsy
necr osis
neo blastic
neo genesis
neo natorum
neo plasm
nephr algia
nephro lith iasis
nephr omento pexy

nephr oncus
nephro ptosis
nephro scler osis
nephro tresis
nesidio blast
nesidio ectomy
nesto therapy
neur a praxia
neur a sthenia
neur iatry
neuri lemm oma
neuro cladism
neuro clonic
neuro glia
neuro hypo physis
neuro lept an algesia
neuro mittor
neuron itis
neurono phage
neur onyma
neuro pil
neuro pile
neuro pro basia
neuro rrhaphy
neuro status
neuro tagma
neuro tmesis
neuro trosis
neutro penia
neutro phil
nevo lip oma
noci ceptive
noct ambulation
nocti phobia
noct uria
nomo graph
nomo topic
normo capnia

normo glyc aemia
normo kal aemic
noso chthono graphy
noso comial
noso nomy
noso poietic
nost algia
nosto mania
not algia
noto chord
nulli parous
nyct algia
nyct al opia
nycto hemeral
nycto typhl osis
nyct uria
nympho mania
nymph oncus

O

ob duction
ochlo phobia
ochro meter
ochro nosis
oculo gyric
oculo motor
odonto iatria
odonto prisis
odonto seisis
odonto tripsis
odyno meter
odyno phagia
oesophago coel
oesophago myo tomy
olecran arthro cace
oleo resis
olfacto meter

olig aemia
oligakis uria
oligo cyt haemia
oligo hypo meno rrhoea
oligo posia
olig uria
oment ectomy
omento pexy
omento tomy
omo clavicular
omo hy oid
omo phagia
omphal elc osis
omphalo chorion
omphalo mes enteric
onco cyto genic
onco cyt oma
onco thlipsis
oneir ana lysis
oneiro genic
oneir ogmus
onomato poiesis
onych auxis
onycho gryp osis
onycho madesis
onycho schizia
onycho tillo mania
oo cephalus
oo cyesis
oo phor ectomy
oo phoro salping ectomy
oo rhodein
ophio tox aemia
ophry osis
ophthalmo phthisis
ophthalmo tono meter
ophthalmo trope
opistho tonus

opsi algia
opsi uria
opso clonia
opsono philic
opsono phoric
opto metry
orbito coelo plasty
orbito nasal
orchid ectomy
orchido pexy
orchi oscheo cele
orchio scirrhus
orchio scirus
oro pharynx
oro rrhoea
oro therapy
ortho crasia
ortho dentine
ortho dia scope
ortho myxo virus
ortho paedics
orth opsia
orth optics
ortho static
orthri opsia
osche itis
oscheo coel
osche oncus
osmo ceptor
osmo dys phoria
osphy arthr osis
osphyo myel itis
osphyo tomy
osseo apo neur osis
osseo fibrous
ossi form
oste ec topia
oste itis

osteo camp
osteo chondral
osteo petr osis
osteo poikil osis
osteo por osis
osteo tylus
ot algia
ot itis
oto lith
oto rhino logy
oto rrhagia
oto scler osis
ot osteon
oxy cephaly
oxy desis
ozo stomia

P

pachy blepharon
pachy colpismus
pachy tene
paed arthro cace
paed erasty
paed iatric
pago plexia
palato plegia
paleo pallium
paleo patho logy
pali lalia
palin dromia
palin opsia
palin phrasia
pall aesthesia
pallido tomy
pampini form
pan agglutination
pan arter itis

pan creas
pan creato pathy
pan demic
pant hodic
panto graph
papill oedema
papillo eryth aema
papill oma
papulo pustular
para bi osis
para centesis
para colp itis
para ec crisis
par algesia
para metrium
para mnesis par aphia
para phim osis
par apsis
parasit aemia
parasiti cide
para tenon
para thyr oid
para typh oid
par otid ectomy
par oxysm
parturi facient
parvo virus
patho crine
patho gnomonic
pechy agra
pecten osis
pectini form
pedicul osis
pedo graph
pedo meter
pelo haemia
pel oid
pelo therapy

penni form
pentos uria
peo ectomy
peo tillo mania
per foration
peri acinal
peri aden itis
peri kymata
perineo coel
perineo rrhaphy
perineo vaginal
peri por itis
peritoneo clysis
periton itis
per meate
pero cormus
pero melus
peron arthr osis
per os
per spiration
per tussis
pes anserinus
petri faction
petro mast oid
phaco erysis
phaco metachoresis
phago cyte
phak itis
phak omat osis
phall an eurysm
phall oncus
phallo rrhoea
phanero genic
pharmaco genic
pharmaco genetic
pheno type
pheno zygous
phleb ectomy

phleb em phraxis
phleb itis
phlebo stasis
phlogo cyte
phlycteno therapy
phoco melia
phono cardio gram
phos genic
phos phene
phos phorus
phot algia
photo phobia
phragmo plast
phren algia
phren em phraxis
phrenico ex eresis
phricto pathic
phryno derma
phryno lysin
phyco myc osis
phymat oid
physali phorous
physo coel
physo metra
physo pyo salpinx
phyto ana phylacto gen
pia mater
pies aesthesia
piez aesthesia
pilo cystic
pilo erector
pil osis
pimel oma
pimel uria
pino cyt osis
pino some
pion aemia
piri form

pisi form
pithec anthrop oid
pityr iasis
plagio cephaly
planti grade
plasm aphaeresis
plasma soma
plasmo lysis
platy basia
platy cnemia
platy rrhine
pleio chlor uria
pleio karyo cyte
pleion ectic
pleion oste osis
pleo cyt osis
pleo morphic
plesio morphic
plethysmo graph
pleur algia
pleuro bronch itis
pleur odynia
plexi form
plexi meter
pneumato cardia
pneumo byssin osis
pneumo coni osis
pneumon aemia
pnoeo gaster
pnoeo scope
pod agra
pod iatrist
pogon iasis
poikilo blast
poikilo thymia
polio dys plasia
polio encephal itis
polio myel itis

polio thrix
pollaki dipsia
pollaki uria
poly cyt haemia
polyp osis
poly saccharide
pompholy haemia
pono graph
ponto cerebellar
poro coel
porphyrin uria
porta caval
porta hepatic
post cibal
posth itis
post mortem
post prandial
pragmat a gnosia
pragmat a mnesia
pre eclampsia
pre ganglionic
presby acusis
presby cardia
presbyo phrenia
presby opia
primi gravida
pro catarxis
procto clysis
procto cysto tomy
procto sigm oid itis
pro dromal
pro gestin
pro karyote
proli gerous
pro paedeutic
pro phylaxis
proprio ceptor
pro ptosis

pro sector
pros encephalon
pro stato rrhoea
pro stato vesicul itis
pros thesis
prot an opia
proteo lysis
proto plasm
prot zo osis
pro traction
psamm oma
psammo therapy
pseudo angina
pseudo cyesis
psittac osis
psomo phagia
psor iasis
psycho metric
psycho somatic
psychro aesthesia
psychro philic
pteryg oid
ptomain aemia
ptom atropine
ptyal agaogue
ptyalo lith
pub arche
pubo femoral
pudend agra
puer peral
puli cide
puncti form
purpuri ferous
py aemia
py arthr osis
py ec chysis
pyel ectasis
pyel itis

pyelo graphy
pyelo ileo cutaneous
pyelo plication
pykno lepsy
pykno meter
pykn osis
pyle phleb itis
pyloro plasty
pyo calyx
pyo chezia
pyo nephr osis
pyo ptysis
pyren aemia
pyreno lysis
pyreto gen
pyreto therapy
pyrexo genic
pyro nyxis
pyro toxin

Q

quadri ceps
quadri gemina
quadri plegia
quadru ped
quintus

R

radicul itis
radiculo medullary
radio auto graphy
radio carpus
radio odontic
rare faction
re calcitrant
recto col itis

recto labial
recto vesicular
re flex
reno graphy
resti brachium
resti form
retino blast oma
retro peri toneal
retro placia
retro spondyl olisthesis
rhabdo my oma
rhabdo virus
rhachio campsis
rhachio chysis
rhachi schizis
rheumat oid
rhin en chysis
rhino canth ectomy
rhino phyma
rhitid ectomy
rhitido plasty
rhiz odon trypy
rhizo tomy
rhod opsin
rube facient

S

Saccharo mycetes
sacr arthro genic
sacro iliac
sacro lumbar
salping ectomy
salping em phraxis
salpingo oo phor ectomy
salpingo stomy
sanio serous
saponi fication

sapr aemia
sarco blast
sarc oid osis
sarco lemma
satyr iasis
scalari form
scaleno tomy
scapho cephaly
scaph oid
scapul algia
scapulo pexy
scat aemia
scato logy
scato philia
scel algia
schisto coelia
schisto glossia
schisto som iasis
schisto somi cide
schiz axon
schizo gony
schiz oid
schizo trichia
scirrh oma
scler itis
sclero corneal
sclero dactyly
scler osis
scolec oid
scoli osis
scol opsia
scopo philia
scoto chromo gen
scoto phobia
sebo rrhoea
sec odont
seismo cardio graphy
selen odont

semini ferous
semi per meable
septic aemia
septico py aemia
sero fibrous
sero hepat itis
sero purulent
seros itis
sero tonin
sesam oid
seti ferous
siagon agra
sial aden itis
sial agaogue
sialo semio logy
sidero cyte
sidero penia
sider osis
sigm oid
sigm oido stomy
silic osis
sinus itis
sinus oid
sito mania
sito toxic
skia gram
skia scope
somato logy
soma tome
somato megaly
somn ambulism
somni facient
somni ferous
sono graph
sono meter
sopori fic
span aemia
spano pnoea

spasmo lytic
spectro graph
spectro photo meter
spermat em phraxis
spermato coel ectomy
spermato zoon
spermi cidal
spermio genesis
spermio tele osis
spermo phleb ectasia
sphacelo derma
sphen oid
spheno parietal
spheno tresia
sphingo lipid
sphingo myelin
sphygmo cardio graph
sphygmo mano meter
sphyr ectomy
spiro gram
spiro scope
splanchnic ectomy
splanchno coel
splanchno micria
splen itis
spleno caval
spleno rrhaphy
spodo genous
spodo phorous
spondyl arthr cace
spondyl ex arth osis
spondyl olisthesis
sporo trich osis
staphyl aemat oma
staphylo kinase
steato pygia
steato rrhoea
stell ectomy

steno bregmatic
steno crotaphia
sterco bilin
sterco lith
stereo cilium
stereo iso meric
stere opsis
stereo taxis
sterno clavicular
sterno cleido mast oid
steth acoustic
steth algia
stetho myos itis
stetho scope
sticho chrome
stoma cace
stomat itis
stomato gloss itis
stomato menia
strepto bacillus
strepto mycin
Strepto thrix
strongyl osis
strum ectomy
styl oid
sub arachn oid
sub jacent
sub scapular
sudori fic
sudori parous
sui cide
super ego
super natant
supra choroid
supra epi trochlear
supra xiphoid
surdi mute
sus tentaculum

syc osis
sym ballo phone
sym bi osis
sym mela
sym phyo genetic
sym physis
syn adelphus
syn apse
syn chysis
syn clitism
syn cope
syn drome
syn echia
syn ophrys
synovio blast
synov itis
syringo coel
syringo myelia

T

tabo paresis
tachy phasis
tachy pnoea
tachysto scope
taenia fuge
talipo manus
tarso meta tarsus
tarso plasty
tel angi ectasis
tel encephalon
telo lemma
ten odynia
tenon itis
teno plasty
tenot agra
teno tomy
terato logy

terat oma
tetra dactylous
tetra logy
tetra stich iasis
thalass aemia
thel arche
thele plasty
thel itis
thermo genesis
thermo labile
thio genic
thoraco centesis
thoraco pagus
threpso logy
thromb ang itis
thrombo arter itis
thrombo phleb itis
thym ectomy
thymo genic
thymo leptic
thyro glossal
thyr oid ectomy
thyro toxic osis
thyro tropic
tibio fibular
tomo graphy
tono meter
topo graphy
torti collis
tox aemia
toxico logy
tox oid
toxo plasm osis
trache itis
trachelo cyll osis
trachelo cyrt osis
tracheo schizis
tracheo stomy

trach oma
trachy phonia
trago maschalia
trago phonia
trago podia
trans lucent
trans parietal
trans sudate
trans vestism
traumato pyra
trepho cyte
Trepo nema
tri ad
tri ante brachia
trich iasis
trich nod osis
Tricho monas
tri gastric
tri gonus
tri nomial
trio cephalus
tri onym
tri otus
triphth aemia
tripl opia
tri stichia
tromo mania
tromo phonia
tropho blast
tropho therapy
Trypano soma
tubercul osis
tuberculo static
tubi ferous
tubo peri toneum
tubulo acinar
tubulo rrhexis
turbin ectomy

tyl ectomy
tympan itis
tympano hyal
typhl itis
typhlo diclid itis
typhl osis
typhlo tomy
tyr emesis
tyr oma
tyro toxin

U

ul algia
ul a trophy
ulcero granul oma
ul eryt haema
ule gyria
ul itis
ulo cace
ul oid
ultra sonic
uni ceps
uni cornus
uni parous
ur a cratia
ur aemia
ur agogue
uranisco chasma
uranisco plasty
urano plasty
urano plegia
urano staphylo plasty
urcei form
urea poiesis
ureter ectasis
uretero colo stomy
uretero phlegma

uretero pyel itis
uretero py osis
urethr em phraxis
urethr eurynter
urethro phyma
urethro staxis
urino crisia
urino dochium
ur odynia
uro flavin
uro glaucin
uro haematin
uro kinetic
ur oncus
uro rubino gen
uro stea lith
utero cervical
uter odynia
utero tropic
uve itis
uveo mening itis
uvi form
uvula ptosis
uvul itis
uvulo ptosis

V

vagin itis
vagino perineal
vago tomy
vago tonia
vago tropic
varici form
varico cele
varico coel
varic oid
varico tomy

varic ula
variol oid
vas deferens
vaso graphy
vaso neuro pathy
vector cardio graphy
veneni ferous
vene plexus
venereo logy
vene section
veno clysis
veno graphy
ventriculo metry
ventricul ostium
vermet oid
vermi cide
vermi fuge
vermin osis
vesico stomy
vesico umbilical
vesicul ectomy
vesicul itis
vesiculo tomy
vibrio cidal
vibri osis
villi kinin
viri potent
vir oid
viro logy
viru cide
viscero ptosis
viscero tropic
visco meter

vitr ectomy
vitreo dentine
vivi section

X

xanth elasma
xantho chromia
xanth odontous
xantho phyll
xanth opsin
xen en thesis
xeno dia gnosis
xeno menia
xero cheilia
xero mycteria
xer ophthalmia
xero phobia
xipho costal
xiph oid
xipho pago tomy

Z

zelo typia
zesto cautery
zonulo lysis
zoon osis
zosteri form
zygo maxillary
zymo gen
zymo lysis
zym osis

Section 3

The Greek and Latin equivalents of English terms used in Section 1

Related words have been included, while the meanings of some words have been greatly modified since classical times. Such change are indicated by an asterisk. In most cases the changes involve an extension of the original meaning to suit new circumstances. Further information is given in Section 1.

Words borrowed from antiquity ...
are not without their delight sometimes.
For they have the authority of years.

Ben Johnson

A

abdomen	G	Coilia
	L	Venter
abnormal	G	Allotrios [Allos – another]
		Para
	L	Malus
abortion	G	Ectrosis
above	G	Hyper
	L	Supra, super
abscess	G	Empyema [Empyeo – to suppurate]
	L	Absessus
absence	G	A, an
		Eremos [Eremia – a desert]
abundance	G	Baros
accelerate, to	L	Celero
access	L	Aditus [Adeo – to go, or, to come to]
accessible	G	Batos [Baino – to step, stand]
accident	G	Symptoma [Sympipto – to fall together, collapse]
acetic		See *acid.*
ache, physical or mental	L	Dolor [doleo – to suffer pain]
acid	G	Oxys
	L	Acetum
acne	G	Of controversial origin; either from **achne**, or from **acme.**
acorn	G	Balanos – also barnacle, necklace fastener, suppository.
	L	Glans, glandula (dim.)
action	L	Actus
activity	G	Ergon [Ergozomai – to labour, work at]
		Praxis [Prasso – to be busy with, practise, effect]
actor	L	Histrio [Possibly connected with the Greek *istriana,* tatooed masks used to imitate the faces of Scythians, barbarians from the north east]
acute	G	Oxys [Oxyno – to make sharp, pointed, acid; to become acutely painful]
addition	G	Prothesis

adhere, to	G	**Hizano** – also, to make to sit, or, to settle down in one place.
adhesion	G	**Synecheia**
adhesive	G	**Ixos** – also, birdlime made from mistletoe berries, used to catch birds.
adjacent (structures)	L	**Adnexus** [**Ad** – to, and **nexus** – something connecting or binding things together]
adult	L	**Pubes** – signs of adulthood because of the growth of (pubic) hair. Later used of the parts of the body on which this hair grows. [**Pubesco** – to become adult]
again	G	**An, ana**
against	G	**Anti** **Enantios** – also, contrary, opposite.
	L	**Contra**
agitated (movement)	G	**Clonos** [**Cloneo** – to be agitated, wild, tumultuous]
aid	L	**Adjuvans**
aim at, to	L	**Peto** [Related to **petomai** (G) – to fly, dash, dart and to **pipto** (G) – to fall, fall upon]
air	G	**Aer** – originally mist or haze, later air. **Pneuma** – used for both atmospheric air, and breath, respiration and odour. Also used for spirit and divine inspiration.
alien	G	**Allotrios** [**Allos** – another]
alike	G	**Homoios, homos.** These two roots have become mixed up in English so that they are often treated as synonyms. The former meant alike in the sense of being of equal status, of equal magnitude, equally matched. The latter emphasised the joint ownership of something, of being two of a kind, having like properties or characteristics. The distinction between these two roots remains of value and should not be lost.
alive	L	**Vivus**; also **vivos** [**Vivo** – to live, be alive]
all	G	**Pas; panta** (gen.). **Pan-** is the combining form used in medical words.
almond	G	**Amygdale** – also, tonsil.

alongside	G	Para
alteration	G	Amoibe
amber	G	Electron. This also meant an alloy of gold and silver, and is connected with the word elector, the gleaming sun.
amnion	G	Amnion
among	G	Epi
	L	Inter
ancestors	L	Atavi
ancient	G	Palaios, paleos
angle	G	Gonia
animal	G	Zoon
ankle	G	Arthron. Used of many other joints, e.g., of neck and limbs, and also voice articulation. [Arthroo – to fasten by a joint, make articulate]
anoint, to	G	Aleipho [Aleipsis – anointing]
anus	G	Proctos
anvil	L	Incus
ape	G	Pithecos
aperture	L	Aditus [Adeo – to go, to come to]
appearance	G	Opsis. See *sight*.
	L	Facies – also, character or nature of something.
appendage	G	Prosthesis
	L	Adnexus
		Appendix
appetite	G	Orexis [Orego – to stretch, reach out for something]
approach, to	L	Advenio [ad – to, and venio – to come]
arch	L	Arcus; fornix. Both had similar meanings: an arch, a vault; even an arched door-way, sometimes used as a euphemism for a brothel.
arm	G	Brachion
	L	Bracchium (sometimes misspelled with one 'c'.) Both were used to refer to the whole arm, but both referred strictly to only the upper arm. The upper and lower arm were differentiated by their own terms – see below.
arm, lower	G	Olene, pechys

	L	**Ulna.** These words meant the arm from the elbow to the wrist, and particularly the ulna bone. **Olene** could include the hand too, but primarily this word meant a bend, a corner or crook, and thus the elbow. **Pechys** was also used to denote the distance between the point of the elbow and the tip of the little finger, i.e., a cubit.
arm, upper	G	**Brachion. Omos** was also used, although it also meant the shoulder.
	L	**Bracchium, umerus.** The latter, like **omos**, originally meant the shoulder but later was used for the upper arm and acquired an initial 'h' to make it humerus.
armpit	G	**Marchale**
around	G	**Peri**
	L	**Circum**
arouse, to	G	**Erethizo** – also, to rouse to anger, provoke to curiosity, to be quarrelsome. [**Erethismos** – irritation, stimulation, provocation]
arrangement	G	**Tagma, taxis** [**Tasso** – to draw up in order or array, place in order or position] **Thesis** – also, deposit (of money) pledge, situation. [**Tithemi** – to place, put]
arrow	L	**Sagitta**
artery	G	**Arteria.** This also was used for the trachea and bronchiae, as well as the ureter, but not for veins. See *bloodvessel.*
articulate, to	G	**Arthroo** [**Arthron** – a joint; **arthrosis** – a connexion or articulation; **arthriticos** – gout, arthritis]
articulation	L	**Articularis**
ashes	G	**Spodos** – also, the ashes of mourning, and the oxides of some metals.
	L	**Cinis**
assuage, to	L	**Lenio** – also, to calm down. [**Lenis** – gentle, mild; **lenitas, lenitudo** – gentleness, smoothness]
assault	G	**Horme** [**Hormao** – to start, rush, attack]
assess	G	**Docimasia** [**Docimazao** – to assess, test, examine]

astringent	G	**Stypteria**; substances containing alum or ferrous sulphate. [**Stypticos** – astringent]
asymmetric	G	**Plagios**
attack	G	**Horme** [**Hormao** – to start, rush, attack]
auger	G	**Trypanon**; a boring tool used by carpenters and a trepan used by surgeons. [**Trypao** – to bore, pierce]
away	L	**A, ab**
away from	G	**Apo**
	L	**A, ab**
		De
axilla	G	**Marchale**
axiom	G	**Axioma** – also honour, rank, suitable, self-evident.
axis	G	**Axon**
	L	**Axis**
axis vertebra	*G	**Stropheus**

B

babble, to	G	**Laleo** [**Lalia** – talk, chat, discussion]
back	G	**Noton** – also, a wide surface.
		Opisthen – towards the rear; but also the hereafter, i.e., in the future. [**Opistho** – backwards]
	L	**Dorsum**, similar to **noton**.
		Tergum, similar to **opisthen**.
backwards	G	**Palin** – associated with returning to or from a place.
	L	**Retro**
bad	G	**Cacos**
		Dys
	L	**Malus**
bald, to be	G	**Madao** [**Madesis** – loss of hair]
bald patches	G	**Alopex** – a fox, hence mange.
band	G	**Lemniscos** – also, a ribbon to hold a chaplet round the head.
	L	**Fascia** – also, a girth, girdle.
		Taenia
bandage	G	**Lemniscos**
	L	**Fascia**

		Taenia
		Pannus – also, a rag, fillet of cloth.
barb	G	**Oncos** – a barb of an arrow.
bark	L	**Cortex** – also, rind; shell.
barley (seed)	L	**Hordeum**
barrier	L	**Obex** [**Obicio** – to throw something in the way: **ob** – before and **iacio** – to throw]
		Saeptum [**Saepio** – to surround, confine]
base	G	**Basis** – also, a step, order, pedestal, foundation. [**Baino** – to step]
	L	**Fundus** [**Fundo** – to found]
basin	G	**Pella**
	L	**Pelvis**
bath or bathing place	L	**Balneum, balineum**
bay	L	**Sinus** – also a dip, curve or fold in the ground; a garment; the coastline.
beak	G	**Coracoeides** – also, like a raven.
		Corone – also, anything hook-shaped: a door-handle, tip of a bow, etc.
	L	**Rostrum** – also, the prow of a boat; gnawing mouth-parts.
beam	G	**Zygon** – also, a yoke, balance beam, yard-arm.
		Actin, actis – also, spoke (of a wheel), ray (of light) and hence brightness. [**Actinos** – radial]
	L	**Trabecula** (dim.) [**Trabs** – a beam]
bean	L	**Faba** (the broad bean, *Vicia faba.*)
bear	G	**Phero** – also, to produce, create, acquire; to be borne away or along.
		Phoreo – also, to possess, hold.
	L	**Fero** [as **phero**]
beard	G	**Pogon**
beat, to	L	**Caedo** (**cecidi, caesum**); to cut down, kill. [Not to be confused with **cado**: see *fall*]
		Palpito
beautiful	G	**Calos**
bed	G	**Cline** – also, a couch, bier.
before	G	**Pro**

	L	Ante
		Prae
beget, to	G	Phyo [Physis – origin, nature]
	L	Gigno
begin, to	G	Hormao
	L	Cresco
beginning	G	Arche
		Catarxis [Catarche – beginning, first]
		Genesis
behind	G	Opisthen – towards the rear; but also the hereafter, i.e., in the future.
	L	Retra
belch, to	L	Eructo
belly	G	Coilia
		Gaster, gastros
	L	Venter
below	G	Hypo – also, under, beneath.
	L	Infra, from inferus
belt	G	Zone; zoster – also, a girdle round the hips used by women; a man's belt; shingles; any girldle-like structure.
bend, to	G	Campto
		Clino – also, to cause to incline or recline.
	L	Flecto
beneath	L	Sub
bent	G	Ankylos [Ankyloo – to bend]
		Grypos [Gryps – a griffin, after its hooked beak and talons]
bent backwards	G	Lordos
	L	Supinus
bent forwards	G	Kyphos – also, stooping, hunchbacked.
	L	Pronus
bent inwards	L	Varus
bent outwards	L	Valgus
berry	L	Acinus
best, to be	G	Aristeuo
best quality	G	Proteios [Proteion – the chief rank of an hierarchy and proteuo- to hold first place]

between	G	Meta
	L	Inter
beyond	G	Hyper – also, over.
		Para – also, alongside, from the side of someone.
	L	Trans – also, across, on the other side of something.
		Ultra – also, further than a certain limit.
bile	G	Chole – also, bitterness, anger, repugnance.
	L	Bilis – as chole
bind, to	G	Deo
	L	Ligo
		Stringo
binding	G	Desmos
	L	Adnexus [ad – to, nexus – something connecting or binding things together]
birth	G	Tocos [Ticto – to produce, bring forth]
		Locheia [Lochizo – to lie in wait for, to ambush]
birth, to give	L	Pario
bite	G	Dexis – also, gnawings, pangs, biting jokes. [Dacno – to bite, sting]
biting	G	Odax – gnashing the teeth in rage or death. [Odactazo – to gnaw, bite]
black	G	Melas
	L	Fuscus
blackhead	L	Comedo, comedones (plur.). When expressed, a blackhead was thought to be a little worm which ate the flesh; hence the association with gluttony.
bladder	G	Cystis
	L	Vesica, vesicula (dim.)
blast	G	Physema [Physao – to blow, puff, distend]
	L	Flatus – also haughtiness.
blemish	L	Macula; both physical and moral.
blind	G	Alaos – also, the dead; that which is invisible.
		Amauros – also, dim, without light.
		Typhlos – also, without insight or understanding; hidden; without an inlet, closed up.
	L	Caecus

blindness	G	Scotos – also, gloom, shadows. [Scotizo to be darkened, blinded]
	L	Nox
blink, to	G	Nicto
blister	G	Phlyctaina [Phlyctainoo – to cause blisters]
		Pomphos [Pompholyx – a bubble; pompholyzo – to boil, bubble up]
block up, to	G	Phrasso [Sometimes phratto]
	L	Obturo
blood	G	Haima
		Ichor
	L	Sanguis – also, blood relationship, life-blood, vigour.
bloodvessel	G	Phleps – also, the veins of plants.
bloodshot	G	Hyphaimos – also, suffused with blood; hot-blooded.
bloom, to	G	Antheo
blue, dark blue	G	Cyanos
bluish green	G	Glaucos
bluish grey	L	Griseus
blunt	G	Amblys
blunt, to make	L	Obtundo
boaster	G	Histrio See actor.
boat-shaped	G	Scaphoeides
body	G	Cormos [Ceiro – to cut off, crop, ravage]
		Soma
	L	Caro
		Corpus
body cavity	G	Coilia
boil	L	Furunculus
bolting together	G	Gomphosis [Gomphos – a bolt, bond, fastening]
bolus	L	Bolus
bond	L	Vinculum [Vincio – to bind, tie]
bone	G	Osteon
	L	Os
border	L	Margo
		Limbus – also, a hem, fringe.
boring tool	G	Trypanon

born, to be	L	**Nasor, natus** [Originally **gnatus** as in pregnant; q.v.]
born, prematurely	L	**Abortus**
bosom	G	**Colpos** – also, lap, womb, the bosom of the sea, a valley.
boss (knob)	G	**Omphalos** (the navel)
	L	**Bulla**
		Umbo
both	G	**Amphi, ampho**
		Amphoteros
	L	**Ambo**
bottom	*G	**Basis**
	L	**Fundus**
bow	L	**Arcus** – also, the rainbow, vault.
bow down, to	G	**Campto**
bowels	L	**Omentum**
bowl	G	**Pella**
	L	**Pelvis**
bow-legged	L	**Valgus**
box	L	**Capsa, capsula** (dim.)
boy	L	**Puer**
brain	G	**Encephalos** [**En** – in, and **cephalos** – head]
	L	**Cerebrum, cerebellum** (dim.)
branch	G	**Clados** – also, the laurel branches used in temples.
	L	**Ramus**
branding iron	G	**Cauterion**
break	G	**Clasis**
		Rhegma
	L	**Fragor**
break, to	G	**Clao**
		Rhegnymi, rhegnuo; rhesso
	L	**Frango**
breast	G	**Mastos, mazos.** Used of males and females.
		Sternon – also, the seat of the affections. Males only.
		Stethos – also, as **sternon** but in males and females.

	L	Mamma – as **mastos**.
		Pectus – similar to **sternon**.
breath	G	**Pnoe** [**Pnoeo** – to blow, breathe]
		Physema [**Physao** – to blow, puff, distend]
	L	**Halitus** [**Halo** – to breathe]
breathe, to	L	**Halo**
		Spiro – also, to blow, exhale, be alive.
breathing	G	**Pneuma** – also, blast, wind, flatulence, breath of life [**Pnoeo** – to breathe] See also *air*.
bride	G	**Nymphe**
bridge	L	**Pons, (pontis)**
bright	G	**Lampros**
brimstone	G	**Theion (thion)** – also, associated with lightning and thunderbolts.
bristle	L	**Saeta**
brittle	G	**Krauros**
broad	G	**Eurys** – also, far-reaching, spread wide.
		Plax – also, wide expanse of sea or sky, flat stone, a tombstone.
bronchus	G	**Bronchos** – also, the trachea and throat. The trachea and bronchi were not differentiated. See *neck*.
broth	L	**Jus**
brother	G	**Adelphos** [**Delphys** – a womb. This word was used of both brothers and sisters, although **adelphe** meant just sisters. **Adelphos** also meant colleague, kinsman; also, anything paired e.g., twins]
bruises	L	**Purpura** [Connected with **porphyra**; See *purple*.]
bruise, to	G	**Thlao**
bubble	G	**Pemphix, pemphigos** (gen.)
		Physa [**Physao** – to blow, distend, be puffed up]
		Pompholyx
bucket	L	**Haustrum**
bud	G	**Blastos** [**Blastano** – to sprout, grow, produce]
	L	**Germen**
bulging	G	**Cyrtosis**
bundle	L	**Fascis**. *Fasces* were the sign of the chief magistrates of Rome.

		Sarcina – also, portable luggage, burden.
burn, to	G	Caio
		Phlego – also, to burst into flames, light up, burn with passion.
bursting	G	Rhexis [Rhegnymi – to burst asunder]
buttock	G	Gloutos
		Pyge
	L	Clunis
		Natis

C

c-shaped	G	Sigma. This letter was earlier a semicircle, and only later became s-shaped.
caecum	G	Typhlon [More correctly typhlines or typhilinos – a blind snake, or caecilian]
	L	Caecum
cake	G	Maza
(disc-shaped)		Plakous
	L	Placenta
calamity	G	Ptome [Ptomaticos – subject to epilepsy, the falling sickness]
calf (of leg)	L	Sura
callus	G	Helos
		Porosis [Poroo – to petrify; poros – building stone]
		Sciros. Some early authors had scirros but none scirrhos and the spelling scirrhus should not be used.
		Tylos
		Tyle
	L	Callum
calloused, to be	G	Poroo
canal	L	Canalis, canaliculus (dim.)
capture	G	Airesis [Aireo – to grasp, take]
carbon	G	Carbo
carbuncle	G	Anthrax [This word is connected with anthracoomai – to be burnt to ashes, or to form a malig-

		nant ulcer, but the reason for this association is not obvious]
care for, to	G	**Comizo**
		Therapeuo [**Therapon** – a male attendant, **therapaina** – a female slave]
carcasss	G	**Creas**
		Ptoma – also, the fallen (in battle).
caries	G	**Sphacelos** [Worse than **gangraina;** See *gangrene.*]
carpet	G	**Stroma**
		Tapes, tapetion (dim.).
carry, to	G	**Phero** – also, to produce, create, acquire; to be borne away or along.
		Phoreo – also, to possess, hold.
	L	**Fero** [As **phero**]
		Veho [**vectum**]
carry around, to	G	**Ago** [**Agoge** – carrying away; **agogos** – guiding, drawing forth]
carry away, to	L	**Defero**
		Effero
carry towards, to	L	**Affero**
cartilage	G	**Chondron**
case	G	**Thece**
cat	G	**Ailouros**
catch, to	G	**Agreo** [**Aireo** – to take, grasp, seize]
caul	G	**Amnion**
		Omentum
causation	G	**Aitia** [**Aitios** – culpable; **aitiaomai** – to accuse]
cause, to	L	**Facio**
caustic	G	**Causticos** [Connected with **caio** – to burn and **cauterion** – a branding iron]
cauterize, to	G	**Caio**
cave	G	**Antron**
cavity	G	**Coilia**
	L	**Alveus, alveolus** (dim.)
cell	G	**Cytos**
chafe, to	G	**Thlibo**
	L	**Tero**

chain	L	**Vinculum** [**Vincio** – to tie, bind, restrain]
chain-armour	G	**Streptos**
chamber	L	**Atrium**
		Locus, loculus (dim.)
chamber, inner	G	**Antron**
		Thalame
chance	G	**Symptoma**
change	G	**Amoibe**
change, to	G	**Allasso**
		Ameibo
	L	**Muto**
changeful	G	**Poikilos**
channel	G	**Solen**
	L	**Alveus, alveolus** (dim.)
		Fossa
charcoal	G	**Carbo**
chatter, to	G	**Laleo**
cheek	G	**Genys**
		Melon – a tree fruit such as apple, apricot, peach; things of a similar shape: the cheeks, a girl's breasts, tonsils, etc.
	L	**Bucca**
		Mala
cheese	G	**Tyros**
	L	**Caseus**
chest, a	G	**Thece**
chest, the	G	**Sternon** – also the seat of the affections. Males only.
		Stethos – as **sternon**, but males and females.
	L	**Pectus** – as **stethos**.
child	G	**Gonos**
		Pais
	L	**Puer**
childbirth	G	**Locheia** [**Lochizo** – to lie in wait for, to ambush]
		Tocos [**Ticto** – to produce, bring forth]
chillblain	L	**Pernio, perniones** (plur.)
chimaera	G	**Chimaira**
chin	G	**Geneion**

		Mentum
cicatrix	G	Oule
circle	G	Cyclos – also, ring, wheel, sphere.
	L	Orbis – also, ring, disc.
circular	G	Halos
	L	Orbis
clapping	G	Crotos
cleanse, to	L	Abluo, ablutum
		Purgo
cleansing	G	Catharsis [Cathairo – to purge, cleanse]
clear	G	Delos [Deloo – to manifest, make known]
		Hyalos
		Leucos, leukos
cleavage, cleft	G	Schisis, schisma [Schizo – to split, cleave]
	L	Crena. The derivation of this word is uncertain.
		Hiatus [Hio – to open, gape]
cloak	G	Chlamys. The short mantle used by horsemen, a military cloak.
	L	Palla. A long, wide mantle used by women.
clod	G	Bolos
close (by)	G	Plesios [Plesiazo – to be near, to approach, approximate]
	L	Juxta
close, to	G	Cleio, kleio [Cleis – a bolt. bar, key]
		Myo
		Phrasso [Phrax, phragma – an enclosing structure]
	L	Occludo [Oc (=ob) – at, against and claudo – to close, shut; connected with kleio and cleis (G)]
clot	G	Thrombus
clotted	*L	Grumus
clothing	G	Ependyma
	L	Indusium. Probably an outer garment.
		Tunica. A woollen shirt or tunic worn by both men and women.
		Vestis
club	G	Coryne
club-foot	G	Kyllos
cluster	L	Racemus

clyster	G	**Clyster.** An enema, an injection into the rectum.
coagulation	G	**Pagos, pexis** [Both from **pegnymi** – to make fast]
coal	G	**Anthrax**
		Carbo
cockle	L	**Concha**
cognition	G	**Noesis** [**Noeo** – to apprehend, think, conceive mentally]
coil	G	**Helix**
cold	G	**Cryos**
		Psychros
	L	**Algor** [**Algeo** – to be cold]
colic	G	**Colicos**
	L	**Tormina**
colour	G	**Chroma.** Both this word and **chros** refer to the complexion and thus to the colour of the skin.
column	G	**Cion (kion)**
		Stylos – also, a writing stylus.
comb	L	**Pecten** [**Pecto** – to comb]
combination	G	**Crasis** [**Cerannymi** – to mix, blend, combine together]
come from, to	L	**Advenio** [**ad** – to, and **venio** – to come]
common	G	**Coinos** – also, shared jointly. [**Coinoneo** – to share, act in common with others]
		Homos [Not **homoios**]; See *alike.*
complete	G	**Holos**
complexion	G	**Chroma**
		Chros
concave	G	**Coilos, koilos**
		Lordos
conceive, to	G	**Cyeo, cyo**
	L	**Concipio**
		Gigno
		[**Cyeo** and **gigno** referred only to the physical impregnation and conception of the female; **concipio** referred mainly to mental conception]
concept	G	**Noema** [**Noeo** – to apprehend, think, conceive mentally]
condensation	*G	**Airesis** [**Aireo** – to take, grasp, seize]; See also *catch.*

condition	G	**Hexis, schesis** [**Echo** – to have, possess, hold, keep] **-sis** [A corruption of **iasis** – a remedy; from **iaomai** – to heal, cure, q.v.] **Stasis** [**Histemi** – to set up, to be placed, stand]
cone	G	**Conos**
confusion	G	**Taraxis** [**Tarasso** – to trouble, purge the bowels, stir up]
congealed	G	**Pectos** [**Pegnymi** – to stick or fix something on or in]
congenital abnormality	G	**Ectroma**
connection	G	**Hapsis** [**Hapto, haptomai** – to fasten, bind, take hold] **Synecheia**
	L	**Adnexus**
conspicuous	G	**Delos** [**Deloo** – to make visible, known, to be manifest]
constrict, to	L	**Coarto** [Not **coarcto**]
contact	G	**Haphe** [**Haptomai** – to take hold of]
contain, to	L	**Concipio**
containing	G	**Dochos** [**Dechomai** – to take, receive]
content	G	**Euchyma**
continuity	G	**Synecheia** [**Synecho** = **syn** and **echo**, to hold together, to be continuous]
contraction	G	**Systole** [**Systello** – to draw together, contract]
contradiction	G	**Palin**
convex	G	**Cyrtos**
convey, to	L	**Affero**
convulsion	G	**Spasmos** [**Spao** – to cause convulsions, spasms]
cook, to	G	**Pepsis** [**Pesso** – to soften by heat, cook]
cord	L	**Funis, funiculus** (dim.)
corn	G	**Helos**
cornea	G	**Keras**
corner	G	**Gonia**
corpse	G	**Necros** **Ptoma** – also, the fallen in war.
correct	G	**Orthos**
	L	**Rectus** [**Rego** – to direct, govern]

corrosive	G	Causticos
couch	G	Cline. This was for reclining on at mealtimes as well as a bed. Also, a bier.
cough	L	Tussis
cover, to	*L	Advenio
		Tego
covering	G	Elytron
		Peritonaios
		Thele
	L	Tectum [Tego – to cover]
		Velum
cow	L	Vacca
crab	G	Carcinos
	L	Cancer
crack	G	Rhagas [Rhegnymi – to break apart]
	L	Rima
creation	G	Poiesis [Poieo – to make, create, cause, produce]
creep, to	G	Herpo
	L	Serpo
crescent (-shaped)	G	Meniscos – the diminutive of meis, the lunar crescent.
		Sigma. This letter was earlier a semi-circle and became s-shaped later.
	L	Lunula [Luno – to bend, to form a crescentic shape]
crest	G	Lophos
		Crista
crooked	G	Cyllos
		Plagios [Plazo – to ward off, thwart]
crossing-over	G	Chiasma
cross over, to	L	Decusso
crowd	G	Ochlos
crown	L	Corona
crown of head	L	Vertex [Verto – to turn round]
crush, to	G	Thlao
cuckoo	G	Coccyx. Also, used to refer to the sacrum. The reason for the association with the cuckoo is unclear.

culmination	G	**Telos**
cup (-shaped)	G	**Calyx** [**Calypto** – to hide, conceal]
		Cotyle
	L	**Acetabulum**, originally a special cup for vinegar.
curdled, congealed	G	**Pectos** [**Pegnymi** – to stick or fix something on or in]
cure	G	**Acesis; acos** [Both words are from **aceomai** – to cure, remedy]
cure, to	G	**Iaomai**
cured	G	**Iathenai** [**Iaomai** – to cure]
curve, to	L	**Flecto**
curved	G	**Ankylos** [**Ankyloo** – to bend]
		Grypos [**Gryps** – a griffin, after its hooked beak and talons]
	L	**Flectum** [**Flecto** – to bend, curve]
cushion	L	**Pulvinus**
custom	G	**Nomos**
		Tropos
cut, to	G	**Keiro** – also, to clip, crop, ravage, plunder.
		Schizo – also, to cleave, divide, separate.
		Temno – also, to prune, slaughter, divide.
	L	**Caedo** – also, to murder, slay, hew down.
		Seco – also, to amputate, castrate, divide.
cutting	G	**Tmesis** [**Temno** – to cut]
cycle	G	**Cyclos**
cylinder	G	**Syrinx** – also, the pipes of Pan, shepherd's pipes; something pipe-like, e.g., bronchi in the lungs, veins, the cavity of the spine, underground passages, etc.
cyst	G	**Meliceris** – also a kind of honey-cake. [**Meli** – honey]

D

daily	L	**Diurnus** (not night)
damage	G	**Trauma** [**Traumizo** – to wound]
dance	G	**Choreia** [**Choreuo** – to take part in a joyful celebratory round-dance]

	L	Saltatio [**Salto** – to dance with gestures, as in a pantomime. Related to **salio** – to jump, leap]
dandruff	G	**Pityrisma, pityriasis** – also, scurf; bran, husks of corn.
dark, darkness	G	**Scotos** – also, blindness. [**Scotoo** – to blind, darken, stupefy]
	L	**Fuscus**
		Nox – also, blindness.
dawn, daybreak	G	**Eos**
		Othrios [**Othros** – dawn]
day	G	**Hemera**
deaden, to	L	**Obtundo**
deaf	G	**Kophos** [**Kophao** – to silence, make dumb or deaf]
deafness	L	**Surditas** [**Surdus** – deaf]
death	G	**Thanatos**
decay	G	**Sepsis** [**Sepo** – to make rotten]
	L	**Caries**
deceiving	G	**Planos** – also, wandering, digression. [**Planao** – to lead astray]
decrease, to	G	**Meioo**
deed	G	**Pragma** [**Prasso** – to pass through, experience, effect]
deep	G	**Bathys**
defaecate, to	G	**Chezo**
defaecation	G	**Lapaxis**
defect (congenital)	G	**Ectroma**
defend, to	G	**Alexo**
		Arceo – also, to succour, suffice.
defilement	G	**Myssos**
deformed	G	**Cyllos, kyllos**
delay	L	**Tardus** [**Tardo** – to slow down]
delicate	G	**Leptos** – also, peeled, threshed, narrow, weak, slight. [**lepto** – to peel]
delimit, to	G	**Orizo**
deltoid	G	**Deltoides**
dense	G	**Pycnos, pyknos** [**Pyknoo** – to pack closely, condense, become dense]

departure	G	**Metachoresis**
deposit	L	**Sequestrum**
deprived, to be	G	**Stereo**
depth	G	**Bathos** – also, height.
desire	G	**Epithymia** [**Epithymeo** – to long for, covet]
		Orexis [**Orego** – to entreat, stretch out, grasp at]
development (sudden)	G	**Eclampsis** [**Eclampo** – to shine out suddenly, burst forth]
devour, to	G	**Phagein**
	L	**Voro**
diaphragm	G	**Phren**
diction	G	**Lexis** [**Lego** – to tell, retell, say, speak]
different	G	**Allos** – strictly, one of several.
		Heteros – strictly, one of two.
digest, to	G	**Pepto**, originally **pesso**
digit	G	**Dactylos**
dilate, to	G	**Euryno**
dilation	G	**Ectasis**
dilation, of pupil	G	**Mydriasis**
dim	G	**Amauros**
		Amblys
direction	G	**Tropos**
direction, (to give)	L	**Gubernaculum** [**Guberno** – to steer a ship]
disable, to	G	**Blapto**
disc	G	**Discos**
discharge	L	**Sanies** [**Sanguis** – blood]
disclose, to	L	**Aperio** [**Apertus** – open; **apertum** – an open space]
discourse	G	**Logos** [**Lego** – to tell, retell, recount]
disease	G	**Itis**. See *inflammation*.
		Nosos – also, madness, distress, bane.
	L	**Morbidus** [**Morbus** – disease, sickness]
disgraceful	L	**Pudendus** [**Pudeo** – to be ashamed, to cause shame]
dislocate, to	L	**Luxo** [**Luxus** – dislocated]
disorder, to	G	**Tarasso** [**Taraxis** – confusion; **tarache** – upheaval, disorder, especially of the bowels]

displacement	G	Metoicia
dissolve, to	G	Cheo
		Lyo
distant	G	Tele [Teleo – to fulfil, bring to perfection or completion]
distinct	G	Lampros
distract, to	G	Blapto
distribution	G	Diairesis
district	G	Demos
divide, to	G	Schizo
	L	Findo
divided	G	Dicha [Dis – twice]
divisibility	G	Diairesis
doctor	G	Iatros [Iatrer – masculine; iatria – feminine]
dog	G	Cyon
door	L	Foris [Foras and foris are from fora = thyra (G), a folding door]
		Ostium
dose	G	Dosis
double	G	Diploos
doubly	G	Amphi, ampho
		Dis, dicha
down (hairs)	L	Lanugo [Lana – wool]
downwards	G	Cata
draw, to	L	Traho
drawing	G	Gramme, graphe. Both words are connected with grapho – to write, draw or delineate, but today the former refers to the written record, while the latter refers to the process of obtaining this.
draw together, to	L	Coarto (Not coarcto.)
		Stringo
dream	G	Oneiros [Oneirosso – to dream]
dregs	L	Faex
dried body	G	Skeletos
drink	G	Posis [Pino – to drink]
dripping (blood)	G	Staxis [Stazo – to drop, drip]
droop, to	G	Ptosis

drop, to	L	Cado
dropsy	G	Hydrops – also, aqueous humour, one of the four humours. [Hydor – water]
drowsiness	G	Caros [Caroo – to stun, stupefy]
		Nystagmos [Nystazo – to doze, nod off]
drug	G	Pharmacon
drum	G	Tympanon – also, a solid wheel, roller. [Tipto – to strike]
dry	G	Krauros [Kraura – a fever, and krauroomai – to become parched and dry]
		Xeros – also, withered, lean, arid.
	L	Siccus – also, sound, healthy; thirsty.
duct	G	Solen
dull, to make	G	Amblys
	L	Obtundo
dumb	G	Kophos [Kophao – to silence, make dumb or deaf]
dung	G	Copros – also, dunghill.
		Scor, scatos (gen.).
	L	Stercus [Stercoreus – filthy, foul]
dusky	G	Phaios
dust	G	Conis
		Spodos – also, the ashes of mourning, and the oxides of some metals.
duty	G	Deon
dwarf	G	Nanos

E

ear	G	Ous [Otos – of the ear]
	L	Auris, auricula (dim.) [Audio – to hear]
ear-drum	?	Myringa – of unknown derivation; perhaps from meninx (G) – a membrane. See also *drum*.
ear, external	L	Pinna
earth	G	Chthon – the world rather than soil.
eat, to	G	Phagein
	L	Voro
eczema	G	Eczema [Eczeo – to boil over, break out]
edge	L	Fimbriae

educate, to	G	Paedeuo
effort	L	Nisus, nixus
egg	G	Oon
	L	Ovum
egg-white	L	Albus
egg-yolk	G	Lecithos
elbow	G	Ancon – also, arm, angle or bend. Olecranon. This word is apparently derived from olene, the lower arm, and cranon. The latter is not the same as cranion, the skull, but may be connected with cranos, a helmet.
	L	Ulna
elsewhere	G	Allache [Allos – another]
embryo	G	Blastos [Blastano – to bud, sprout] Embryon
	L	Germen
emission	*G	Ogmos
emit, to	L	Eructo Mitto
emphasis	L	Per
empty	G	Cenos, kenos [Kenoo – to empty] Coilos
	L	Vacuus – also, exempt, lacking something.
empty, to	G	Alapazo
enamel	G	Adamas
	F	Amel
encircling structure	G	Stephanos – also, a crown, wreath. [Stepho – to encircle, put around, crown]
enclosure	L	Claustrum [Claudo – to shut, close, conclude; connected with clavis and cleis]
end	G	Telos [Teleo – to fulfil, bring to perfection or completion]
enema	G	Eniemi. A nutritive enema was also used: "trophimoi clyster". See also clyster.
engrave, to	G	Glypho
engraving tool	G	Xyster [Xeo – to scrape]
enlarge, to	L	Laxo
entire	G	Holos

entrance	L	**Aditus**
		Atrium
		Meatus [**Meo** – to go, pass]
		Ostium
		Porta
		Vestibulum
entry	G	**Endysis** [**Endyo** – to enter, go into; also, to put on, clothe.
epidermis		See *hide, leather.*
equal	G	**Homoios**
		Isos
erupt to		See *to bloom, flower.*
escape	G	**Phyge** [**Pheugo** – to flee, escape]
ethics		See *proper, right.*
evacuation (of bowels)	G	**Lapaxis**
even	G	**Homalos**
evening	G	**Opse, opsi**
event	G	**Climacter** [**Climax** – a ladder, from **clino** – to lean, incline]
		Pragma [**Prasso** – to pass through, experience, effect]
evident	G	**Phaneros** [**Phaino** – to make known, reveal]
evil	G	**Cacos**
examination	G	**Docimasia** [**Docimazo** – to assay, test]
exchange, to	L	**Muto**
excision	G	**Ectome**
excrement	G	**Copros** – also, a dunghill.
		Scor, scatos (gen.)
		Scybalon
	L	**Stercus** [**Stercoreus** – filthy, foul]
exertion	L	**Nisus**
experience, to	L	**Concipio.** Although this verb was primarily concerned with conception in pregnancy, it acquired by transference the connotation of mental conception. It is connected with the verb **nosco** – to get to know, to investigate, which was earlier **gnosco**, and cognate with **gignosco** (G) – to perceive, know.

expert	G	**Gnomon** [**Gignosco** – to know, perceive, think]
explanation	G	**Hermeneia** [**Hermeneusis** – style, expression; **hermeneuo** – to interpret, express, describe]
expression	G	**Phasis** – also, rumour, tidings. [**Pheme** – prophecy, speech]
		Phrasis [**Phrazo** – to point out, declare, advise, perceive]
extend, to	G	**Mecyno** [**Mecynosis** – lengthening]
		Teino
	L	**Tendo**
extension	G	**Diastole**
		Ectasis [**Ecteino** – to stretch out, spread]
extremity	G	**Acros** [**Ace** – a point; **acis** – something pointed, a needle]
exudation	G	**Hidros** [**Hidroo** – to sweat]
		Ichor
	L	**Serum**
exude, to	L	**Fluo**
eye	G	**Ophthalmos**
	L	**Oculus**
eyeball	G	**Glene**
		Logas, logades (plur.) – more correctly, the whites of the eyes.
eyebrow	G	**Ophrys**
eye corner	G	**Canthos**
		Lacus
eye-lash	L	**Cilium.** Originally the eye-lid, later transferred to the eye-lashes.
eyelid	G	**Blepharon**
	L	**Cilium**
		Palpebra [**Palpo** – to touch gently, to coax, flatter]
eyelid eversion	G	**Ectropion**
eyelid rim	G	**Tarsos**

F

face	G	**Opsis.** See *sight.*

Prosopon [**Pros** – from, and **ops, opos** (gen.) –
face, eye, countenance.]

face-down	L	**Pronus**
facial fold	G	**Rhitis** [**Rhytidoo** – to make wrinkled, shrivelled]
faeces	G	**Copros**
		Scor, scatos (gen.)
		Scybalon
	L	**Stercus**
faeces, baby's	G	**Meconium**
fail, to	G	**Hamartano** [**Hamartema** – failure, fault]
fall	G	**Ptosis** [**Pipto** – to fall down; **ptoma** – a fall, fallen body, corpse]
fall, to	L	**Cado**
		Prolabor [**Prolapsio** – a slipping, sliding]
fall down, to	L	**Labor** – also, to work.
fall off, to	G	**Madao**
falsehood	G	**Pseudes**
family	G	**Gone**
famine	G	**Limos**
fast	G	**Tachys, tachistos** (sup.)
	L	**Celer**
fasten together, to	G	**Hapto**
		Pegnymi
fasting	G	**Nestis**
	L	**Jejunus**
fat	G	**Elaion**
		Lipos
		Pimele
		Pion
		Stear
	L	**Adeps** [Related to **aleipho** (G) – to anoint with oil, polish]
		Pinguis
		Sebum
fatigue	G	**Copos**
feather	L	**Penna, pinna**
feeding on	G	**Ereptomai**
feed on, to	G	**Phagein**

feel, to	L	**Sentio** – applies to both physical and mental actions.
female	G	**Thelys** [**Thelyno** – to make feminine]
feminine	L	**Muliebris** [**Mulier** – a woman, wife]
fence	G	**Phrax** [**Phrasso** – to contain, close off]
fermentation	G	**Sepsis** [**Sepo** – to make putrid]
fever	G	**Causos** [**Caio** – to set on fire; **causoo** – to burn fiercely]
		Pyr
		Typhos. One of four types of fever; also, delusion, humbug, vanity.
	L	**Febris** [**Ferveo** – to be boiling hot, to be fiery]
feverish, to be	G	**Pyresso**
few	G	**Oligos**
fibre	L	**Fibra, fibrilla** (dim.).
fibrous structure	G	**Is, inos** (gen.)
fibula	G	**Perone**. See also *pin*.
fickle	G	**Planos** – also, wandering in mind, error, imposter.
fifth	L	**Quintus**
fig	G	**Sycon** [**Sycea** – the fig tree, *Ficus carica*]
file	G	**Xyster**
file, of men	G	**Stichos**
fill full, to	L	**Farcio** [Related to **phrasso** (G) – to close up, fence in]
filling	G	**Enchyma**
filth	G	**Copros**
		Rhypos
fin	G	**Branchion**
		Pinna
fine	G	**Leptos** – also, peeled, thin, weak, slight, subtle, refined.
	L	**Subtilis** – also, discriminating. [**Tela** – a fine web, **texo** – to weave]
finger	L	**Digitus** – also, one sixteenth of a Roman foot, a finger's breadth, approximately 2 cm.
fire	G	**Pyr**

firm	G	**Stereos**, not to be confused with **stereo**.
first	G	**Protos**
	L	**Primus** (superlative of **prior** – before, former.)
fish	G	**Ichthys**
fissure	G	**Rhagas** [**Rhegnymi** – to break apart]
fixation	G	**Pexis** [**Pegnymi** – to fasten together]
fixed	G	**Pagos**
		Pectos – also, planted, compacted, frozen. [Both words are connected with **pegnymi** – to fasten together]
flabby	L	**Flaccus, flaccidus**
flame	G	**Phlox** [**Phlego** – to burn]
		Pyr
flank	G	**Lapara**
	L	**Latus**
flat	G	**Homalos**
		Plax
flax	G	**Linon** – also, anything made of flax: fishing-nets, hunting nets, linen garments.
flayed	G	**Dartos** [**Dero** – to skin or flay animals; to separate by tearing apart]
flea	L	**Pulex**
flee, to	L	**Fugio** [Related to **pheugo** (G) – to flee, take flight]
flesh	G	**Creas**
		Sarx – also, the flesh of fruits.
	L	**Caro** – as **sarx**
flight	G	**Phyge** [**Pheugo** – to flee]
	L	**Fuga** [Related to **phyge** (G) – to flee]
flint	L	**Silex** – also, any hard stone, a rocky crag.
float, to	L	**Nato** [**No** – to swim; related to **neo** (G) – to swim]
floating	L	**Natans** [**Nato** – to float]
flood	G	**Chysis** [**Cheo** – to pour, flow]
flow	G	**Rheuma** [**Rheo** – to flow, run]
flow, to	G	**Rheo**
	L	**Fluo**
flower, to	G	**Antheo**
fluid	G	**Chymos**

flush	G	**Erythema** [**Erythaino** – to paint red, become red, blush]
flux	G	**Rheuma** [**Rheo** – to flow, run]
fly	G	**Myia**
flying	G	**Ptenos** [**Petomai** – to fly]
foetal caul	G	**Amnion**
fold	G	**Ptyx** [**Ptysso** – to fold, double up]
fold, to	L	**Plico** [Related to **pleco** (G) – to twine, plait]
folding double	G	**Diclis** [**Dino** – to make to recline, one thing to lean against another]
following	L	**Posterus, posterior** (comp.)
food	G	**Broma** [**Bibrosko** – to eat]
		Sitos [**Sitizo** – to feed]
		Trophe [**Trepho** – to rear, suckle, feed]
foot	G	**Pous**
	L	**Pes, pedis; pediculus** (dim.)
force	L	**Vis**
forearm		See *arm, lower.*
forehead	G	**Bregma**
		Metopon, metapos
	L	**Frons**
fork	L	**Furca**
form	G	**Eidos** [**Eido** – to see, perceive]
		Morphe [**Morphoo** – to give form to]
		Plasma – also, forgery, affectation. [**Plasso** – to mould, form]
	L	**Forma** [**Formo** – to shape, form]
form, to	G	**Plasso**
	L	**Facio**
fortification	G	**Teichos**
forward	G	**Pro**
foster	G	**Trepho**
foundation	G	**Basis** – also, a step, order, foot, pedestal. [**Baino** – to step]
fourfold	L	**Quadrigeminus**
fox	G	**Alopex**
fracture	G	**Rhegma** [**Rhegnymi** – to break apart]
fracture, to	L	**Frango** – also, to shatter, humble, subdue.

fragment	G	Clasma [Clao – to break]
freckle	G	Ephelis
		Lentigo
freeze, to	L	Gelo
frenzy	G	Lyssa – also, rabies (in dogs).
friable	G	Psathyros
friction	*G	Aliptic, aleipho
fringe	L	Fimbriae
from	G	Apo
		Pros
front, of head	G	Metapon, metapos
frost	G	Cryos
		Pagos [Pegnymi – to fasten together, make rigid]
fruit	L	Pomum – also, a fruit tree.
fruit-stone	G	Pyren – also, hard bone of fishes, grain of frankincense.
full of, to be	G	Bryo
fungus	G	Myces – also, any knobbly-shaped structure, excrescences on trees.
funnel-shaped	L	Infundibulum [Infundo – to pour in]
furrow	G	Ogmos
	L	Stria
		Sulcus
fusion	G	Chysis
		Syzygia

G

gangrene	G	Gangraina – not so severe as sphacelos. See *caries*.
		Sphacelos [Sphacelizo – to mortify, have convulsions]
garment	G	Ependyma. [Epi – on, and endyma – garment] [Endyo – to put clothes on; ependyo – to put on more clothes]
	L	Indusium
		Tunica
		Vestis – also, a blanket, carpet. [Related to esthys (G) – clothing]

gap	G	**Chasma**
gape	L	**Rictus** [**Ringor** – to show the teeth, snarl]
gape, to	L	**Oscito** [**Os** – mouth and **ceio** – to move. Related to **kineo** (G) – to move]
gaping	G	**Cheme** [**Chasco** – to yawn, gape]
gargle	L	**Collutorium** [**Col** – with, and (**ab**)**lutum** – washed]
gas	G	**Aer**
gate	G	**Pyle** – also, customs house, entrance to Hades, a mountain pass, a narrow strait.
	L	**Porta**
gate-keeper	G	**Pyloros** [**Pyloreo** – to keep the gate, act as a warder]
genitalia	G	**Gonos**
		Medea (plural of **medos**)
gentle	G	**Malacos** [**Mallaso** – to make soft, supple]
germ	G	**Blastos**
gill	G	**Branchion**
girdle	G	**Zoster** – a warrrior's belt. [**Cingo** – to surround, encircle]
		Zona, zonula (dim.) – a maiden's girdle. [Related to **zone** (G) – a woman's girdle worn around the hips]
gland	G	**Aden**
		Boubon
		Glandula (dim. of **glans**)
glass, glass-like	G	**Hyalos**
	L	**Vitreus** [**Vitrum** – glass]
gleaming	G	**Glaucos**
glistening	L	**Candidus** – also, lucid, honest, happy [**Candeo** – to glitter, shine]
glue	G	**Colla** [**Collao** – to glue, cement together]
		Glia; gloios
glue together, to	L	**Glutino**
gnash the teeth, to	G	**Brycho, bryco; bryxo** (future tense)
		Mastichao
		Prio [**Prisis** – gnashing of teeth in rage]

go, to	L	Eo [Related to **eimi** (G) – to exist, be]
		Meo
goat	G	**Aix** – usually applied to both males and females.
		Tragos – also, a fish, a kind of sponge, and a plant.
	L	**Hircus**, male and **capra**, female.
gobbet	G	**Psomos**
goitre	L	**Struma**
gold	G	**Chrysos** – also, other precious things, e.g., copper, silver, iron, vestments. This word is associated with high office and dignity.
golden colour	G	**Xanthos**
goose, of a	L	**Anserinus** [**Anser** – a goose]
gout	*G	**Agreo**
		Arthriticos
graceful	G	**Calos, callos**
grain(s)	G	**Athare** [**Atheroma** – a tumour containing gruel-like matter]
		Chondros
		Coccos
	L	**Granus, granulum** (dim.).
grape	L	**Acinus**
		Uva, uvula (dim.).
grapes, bunch of	G	**Staphyle** [Originally spelt staffa or stapha]
	L	**Racemus**
		Uva – also, a swarm of bees.
grasp, to	G	**Hapto**
grasping	G	**Airesis** – also, conduct, religious or philosophical sect, proposal, etc. [**Aireo** – to grasp by the hand, seize, overpower, grasp with the mind]
grate, to	L	**Strideo** [**Stridor** – a creaking, grating noise]
gravel	L	**Calculi** – (dim. of **calx**.)
grease	L	**Sebum** – also, tallow, fat, suet.
great	G	**Megas, megale; megalou** (gen.)
greater	G	**Hyper**
	L	**Supra, super**
great grand-father	L	**Atavis**
green	G	**Chloasma**. This is a corruption of **chlorasma**,

which is the same as **chlorotes**. This means both greenness and yellowness; also, the pale colour of a mixture of gold and silver.

Chloros [**Chloazo** – to be bright green]

grey	G	**Phaios** – a mixture of black and white.

Polios – also, venerable, hoary.

grey matter	*L	**Cinis**
	?	**Griseus**. Of unknown origin.
grief	G	**Ponos** [**Penomai** – to toil, have need of; **peneo** – to be poor]
	L	**Dolor** [**Doleo** – to suffer pain, grieve]
grinding	G	**Trismos, trigmos**
grind, teeth, to	G	**Brycho, bryxo**

Prio [**Prisis** – grinding of teeth in rage]

grip	G	**Haphe** [**hapto, haptomai** – to fasten to, fasten oneself to, grasp]
gripes	L	**Tormina** [**Torqueo** – to twist, wrench]
gritty		**Acervus**. Note: **acervulus** is a late invention and not found in Latin.
groats	G	**Athare** [**Atheroma** – a tumour containing gruel-like matter]
groin	G	**Boubon**
	L	**Inguen**
groove, of lip	G	**Philtron** – also, a love-charm, a spell, love, affection. [**Phileo** – to love, show affection]
grow, to	G	**Auxano**
		Phyo
	L	**Cresco**
growth	G	– **oma**, only as a suffix.

Phyma [**Phyo** – to produce, create, grow]

Physis – also, appearance, natural order, nature, kind, origin.

growth, to promote	G	**Trepho** – also, to thicken a liquid, to be reared (especially during the first five years), cherish, nourish, educate.
guarding	G	**Phylaxis** [**Phylasso** – to keep watch, guard, defend]
gulf	G	**Chasma**

gullet	G	Oesophagos [Oiso – from future tense of **phero** – to carry]
		Stomachos
	L	Faux
gum	G	Mastiche
gums, of teeth	G	Oulon, oula (plur.)
	L	Gingivae
guts(s)	G	Chorde
		Enteron
	L	Ile, ilia (plur)

H

habit	G	Tropos [Trepo – to turn, direct towards]
haemorrhoid	L	Marisca – also, a kind of large fig.
hair	G	Chaite
		Philos – felt used inside shoes or helmets.
		Thrix
	L	Lanugo – the down on plants or on the cheeks.
		Saeta
hair, to cut off one's	G	Keiro
half	G	Hemi
	L	Semis
ham	L	Poples
hammer	G	Sphyra
	L	Malleus, malleolus (dim.)
hand	G	Cheir – also, hand plus arm, arm, paw.
	L	Manus – also, arm, fist (suggesting power).
handle	L	Manubrium [Related to **manus**]
hard	G	Adamas – also, fixed, unalterable.
		Scleros – also, bitter (taste), rigid, austere.
		Stereos
		Trachys – also, uncouth, austere, severe.
hard, to become	G	Poroo
hard skin	G	Sciros
	L	Callosus, callum

hardly	G	**Mogis**. Also spelt **mygis** and **molis** [**Mogeo** – to toil, suffer]
hare	G	**Lagos**
	L	**Lepus**
harm,	L	**Noxa** [**Noceo** – to harm]
harm, to	G	**Blapto**
	L	**Noceo**
hasten, to	L	**Celero**
haunch	G	**Ischion**
have, to	G	**Echo**
head	G	**Cephale**
	L	**Caput** [Related to **cephale** (G) – the head]
head (anterior part)	L	**Sinciput**, opposite to **occiput**.
heal, to	G	**Iaomai**
healed, to be	G	**Iathenai**
healer	G	**Iatros** [**Iaomai** – to heal]
healing	G	**Acesis**
healthy	G	**Hygieia**
heap		**Acervus**. Note: **acervulus** is a late invention and not found in Latin.
		Grumus
hear, to	G	**Acouo**
	L	**Audio**
heart	G	**Cardia** – also, desire, mind, cardia of the stomach.
	L	**Cor** [Related to **cer** (G) – heart]
heartburn	G	**Causos**
heat	G	**Causos** [**Caio** – to set on fire]
		Phlegma. One of the four humours of the body; malignant, angry. [**Phlego** – to burn, inflame]
		Therme, therma – also, feverish heat.
heaviness	G	**Baros** – also, torpor, influence, dignity.
heavy	L	**Gravis** [Related to **barys** (G) – heavy]
hedgehog	G	**Echinos**
heel	L	**Calx**
height	G	**Hypsos** [**Hypsi** – high]
heir	L	**Heres**
helmet	L	**Galea**

hexagonal	L	**Favus.** Note: **faveolus** is a late invention and not found in Latin.
hiccough	L	**Singultus** – also, croaking of raven, dying rales. [**Singulto** – to sob, hiccough, gasp out]
hidden	G	**Cryptos** [**Cryptoo** – to hide, cover over, conceal]
	L	**Occultus** [**Occulo** – to cover, hide]
hide	*G	**Bursa**
		Dartos
		Derma
		Both **dartos** and **derma** are related to **dero** – to flay animals; to separate by tearing apart.
	L	**Corium, corius**
hill	G	**Bounos**
	L	**Grumus**
hinge	G	**Ginglymos** – also, gudgeon pin of a door hinge, clasp, mode of kissing. **Stropheus** – also, the socket in which the gudgeon pin turned, a vertebra. [**Strepho** – to turn, swivel, twist]
hip	G	**Ischeon**
	L	**Coxa**
hippocampus	G	**Hippocampus** [**hippos** – horse, and **campos** – a sea-monster]
hit, to	G	**Plesso**
hold, to	G	**Echo** [to possess] **Ischo** [to retain]
holder	L	**Tenaculum.** This originally meant a pin or fastener, or a writing instrument. **Tenacula** meant forceps. [Both are from **tenax** – holding, gripping. and **teneo** – to hold]
holding back	G	**Cathexis**
hollow	G	**Antron**
		Cotyle
	L	**Alveus, alveolus** (dim.)
		Sinus
		Valles, vallecula (dim.)
hollow, of foot or hand	L	**Vola**

hollow space	G	**Coilos, koilos**
home	G	**Oicos**
home, to go	G	**Nosteo**
honeycomb	G	**Meliceris**
hook	G	**Cleis** – also, key, catch, tongue of a clasp. [**Cleio** – to shut, close. Related to **clavis** (L) – a key and **claudo** (L) – to shut]
		Corone – also, anything hook-shaped.
	L	**Hamus, hamulus** (dim.)
		Uncus
hooked	G	**Grypos**
horn	G	**Ceras, keras**
		Cornu
horny	L	**Corneus**
horrible	G	**Phrictos** [**Phrisso** – to be rough, to bristle (of hair, of a mane, with spears), to shudder at]
hot	G	**Zestos**
house	G	**Oicos**
hub	L	**Modiolus** – also, a drinking cup, a cog, a kind of trepan. [Related to **modius** – a measure]
human	L	**Homo** [Related to **humus** (L) – the soil, earth and **chamai** (G) on the ground]
		Humanus
humidity	L	**(H)umor**
humped	L	**Gibbus** [Related to **kyphos** (G) – hump, and **krypto** (G) – to stoop]
hunch-backed	G	**Cyrtos, cyrtosis**
		Kyphos, kyphosis [**Krypto** – to stoop]
hunger	G	**Limos**
hungry	L	**Jejunus**
hurt, to	G	**Blapto**
	L	**Noceo**

I

I	G	**Ego**
icy	G	**Cryos** – also, frost.
idea	G	**Noema** [**Noeo** – to perceive, apprehend]

image	G	**Eicon** – also, phantom, representation.
	L	**Spectrumo** [**Specio** – to behold. Related to **sceptomai** (G) – to to look about, consider]
imitative	G	**Mimeticos** [**Mimeomai** – to imitate]
immobility (of joints]	G	**Ankylosis**
imperfect	G	**Ateles** [a – not, and **telos** – , complete]
important	G	**Basilicos**; really kingly, royal, choice. [**Basileus** – king, **basileia** – queen]
		Megas, megale, megalou (gen.)
impregnated, to be	G	**Cyeo**
impulse	G	**Horme** [**Hormao** – to begin, start something]
in	G	**En**
incessant movement	*G	**Athetos**
incise, to	G	**Glypho** – also, to carve, engrave [**Glyphe** – a carving]
incline, to	G	**Clino** – also, to cause to incline, to recline.
incomplete	G	**Ateles** [a – not, and **telos** – complete]
increase, to	G	**Auxano**
		Plethyo
	L	**Cresco**
increasing	G	**Ana**
inflame, to	G	**Phlego** – also, to burst into flames, burn with passion.
inflammation	G	**Itis**. See *disease*.
		Phlegma
inheritance	L	**Hereditas**
injure, to	G	**Noceo**
injurious	L	**Malignus** [**Malus** – bad]
injury	G	**Trauma** [**Traumatizo** – to injure]
		Eso
	L	**Intra**
		Intus [Related to **entos** (G)]
		Trosis [**Titrosko** (**troo**) – to wound, damage, kill]
inner part	L	**Medulla** [**Medius** – middle]
inscription	G	**Graphe**

insertion	G	**Enthesis**
inside	G	**Endon, entos**
	L	**Intra**
intention	G	**Gnome** – also, intelligence, inclination, verdict.
intermediate	G	**Mesos (mese, meson)**
internal organ	G	**Splanchnon** – also, the seat of the feelings.
	L	**Viscus, viscera** (plur.)
interpretation	G	**Hermeneia [Hermaneusis** – style, expression; **hermaneuo** – to interpret, express, describe]
interval	G	**Bathmos [Baino** – to step, walk]
		Diastema
intestinal obstruction	G	**Eileos** – also used with reference to jaundice, scurvy, and some other diseases.
intestine(s)	L	**Ile, ilia** (plur.)
		Jejunum
into	G	**Eso**
	L	**In**
involuntary	G	**Aecon, acon**
	*	**Athetos**
iron	G	**Sideros** – also, hard things, and things made of iron.
irrigation bucket	L	**Haustrum**
irritate, to	G	**Erethizo** – also to rouse to anger, provoke to curiosity. [**Erethismos** – irritation, stimulation, provocation]
island	L	**Insula**
islet	G	**Nesos, nesidion** (dim.)
itch	G	**Psora, psoros**
	L	**Prurigo [Purio** – to itch]
ivory	L	**Eburneus, eburnus**

J

jaundice	G	**Icteros**
jaw	G	**Gnathos, gnathmos** – also, the cheek.
		Genys
	L	**Mandibula [Mando** – to masticate]

jaw bone	G	**Siagon, siegon**
	L	**Mala, maxilla** (dim.)
jealousy	G	**Zelos** – also, pride, glory. [**Zeloo** – to be jealous, envy; also to emulate, praise].
join, to	G	**Arthroo** [**Arthron** – a joint; **arthrosis** – a connexion or articulation; **arthriticos** – gout, arthritis] **Hapto**
	L	**Jungo** – also, to connect, couple. [**Jugum** – a pair, couple; a yoke or beam]
joining	L	**Artus, articulus** (dim.); **articularis**
joint	G	**Arthron** [**Arthroo** – to join] **Gonia**
joint, fluid of	G	**Synovialis**
joint, immobility of	G	**Ankylosis** – also, tongue-tied; adhering eyelids. [**Ankyloo** – to bend, to be crooked]
judgement	G	**Gnome** – also, intelligence, inclination, verdict.
jug	G	**Aryter, arytaina**
	L	**Urceus, urceolus** (dim.)
jug-handle	G	**Ous**
juice	G	**Chylos**
	L	**Jus** **Sucus, succus** – also, flavour, nectar, sap, vigour.

K

keel	L	**Carina**
kernal	G	**Karyo** **Pyren** – also, the hard bone of fishes, grain of frankincense; a kind of gem-stone.
	L	**Nucleus** (dim.) [**Nux** – a nut]
key	G	**Cleis**
	L	**Clavis**
kick, to	L	**Calcitro**
kidney(s)	G	**Nephros**
	L	**Renes**
kill, to	L	**Caedo**
kind	G	**Eidos** **Genos, genna**

	L	**Genus**
knead, to	G	**Masso** – also, to press into a mould, especially when making certain cakes.
knee	G	**Gony**
	L	**Genus** [Related to **gony** (G)]
knee, back of	L	**Poples**
knob	G	**Condylos**
		Coryne
		Tylos
	L	**Furunculus**
knock, to	G	**Ballo**
		Copto
		Plesso
	L	**Pello** – also, to impel, move, drive away.
knock-kneed	L	**Varus**
knot	G	**Ganglion**
		Tylos
	L	**Nodus** – also, conundrum, entanglement, perplexity.
knowledge	G	**Gnosis**
known	G	**Gnotos**

L

labour pains	L	**Nisus**
lack	G	**Eremos** [**Eremia** – a desert]
		Penia [**Peneo** – to be poor]
		Spanis, spanios, spanos [**Spanizo** – to be scarce, in want]
lack, to	G	**Leipo** [**Leipsis** – failure, lack]
lacking position	G	**Athetos**
ladder	L	**Scala**
lake	L	**Lacus** – also, a basin, trough, vat.
lame, to be	L	**Claudico** [**Claudus** – limping]
languid	L	**Flaccidus, flaccus**
large	G	**Macros**
larger	G	**Hyper**
	L	**Supra, super**

late	G	Opse, opsi
latent	G	Cryptos – also, deep-seated.
lattice-work	L	Cancelli [Cancello – to form a trellis-work]
laughter	G	Gelos [Gelao – to laugh, laugh at, deride]
	L	Risus [Rideo – to laugh, laugh at]
law	G	Nomos
lawless	G	Athetos
laws of optics, pertaining to	G	Opticos
lay waste, to	G	Tribo
layer	L	Lamina
lead, to	G	Ago
	L	Duco
leaf, leaflet	*L	Lamina, lamella
lean on, to	G	Skepto [Skepsis – pretext, excuse, pretence]
leap, to	G	Pedao
	L	Subsulto [Subsilio – to leap, spring up]
leather	L	Bursa
		Corium, corius
leave, to	G	Leipo
leaven	G	Zyme [Related to zo – to live, quicken]
left hand side	G	Aristeros [Opposite to dexios – right hand side]
leg	G	Cneme – the shank between knee and ankle; also, the internode of a plant stem, spoke of a wheel.
		Scelos
legume	G	Lathyros [Possibly *Lathyrus sativus*]
	L	Faba [The broad bean, *Vicia faba*)
length	G	Mecos [Related to macros – large]
lengthen, to	G	Mecyno
lentil	G	Phacos, phakos
	L	Lens
lessen, to	G	Meioo
let go, to	G	Hiemi, (hienai) – also, to send, throw, hasten. The suffix -esis is derived from this verb.
let loose, to	G	Regnymi (rhegnuo, rhesso)
level	G	Homalos
lichen	G	Leichen
life	G	Psyche

Vita [**Vivo** – to live, be alive]

life, mode of	G	**Bios**
light	G	**Leucos, leukos**

Phos, correctly spelt **phaos, photos** – also, day-light, a day, window, light of God, mental illumination.

	L	**Lumen**

Lux [**Luceo** – to shine, be bright]

lighten, to	L	**Fulgeo, fulguro, fulmen** (originally **fulgmen**), **fulgino**
lightning (flash)	L	**Fulgor, fulgur, fulmineus**
likeness	G	**Eidolon** – also, a phantom, fancy. [**Eido** – to see, perceive]
limb	G	**Melos** – also, musical phrase, song, melody.
limp, to	L	**Claudico** [**Claudus** – limping]
line	L	**Linea** – also, a linen thread, a plumb-line, a boundary. [**Linum** – flax, linen]
linen	G	**Linon** – also, anything made of linen; fishing-nets, hunting nets, linen garments.
linen thread	G	**Byssos**
	L	**Linea**
linked together	G	**Gomphosis** [**Gomphos** – a bolt, bond, fastening]
		Streptos
lip	G	**Cheilos**
	L	**Labia, labium**
liquid	G	**Hygros**
	L	**Sucus, succus** – also, flavour, nectar, sap, vigour.
liquify, to	G	**Cheo**
listen, to	G	**Acouo**
	L	**Ausculto** – also, to overhear, listen secretly.
little	G	**Micros**
	L	**Parvus**
lively	L	**Vegetus** [**Vegeo** – to quicken, liven up, excite]
liver	G	**Hepar**
	L	**Jecur** – also, the seat of the passions.
living	L	**Vivus** [**Vivo** – to live, be alive]
lizard	L	**Lacerta, lacertus**
loin muscles	G	**Psoa; psoai, psoas**, (plur.)

look, to	G	**Blepo**
		Scopeo – also, to behold, watch for.
looped-shaped	L	**Ansa**
loose	G	**Manos** – also, infrequent, spreading. [**Manoo** – to make loose, porous]
	L	**Patulus** – also, spreading. [**Pateo** – to be open, lie open. Related to **patannymi** (G) – to be spread out, wide open]
loosen, to	G	**Chalao** [**Chalasis** – loosening, relaxation]
		Lyo
loss	G	**Zemia** [**Zemioo** – to cause loss, to damage, penalize, fine, punish]
love, to	G	**Phileo**
lover	G	**Erastes** [**Eramai** – to love sexually, passionately]
luminous, to be	L	**Luceo**
lump	*G	**Embolus**
		Thrombos – also, curd, nipple. [**Thrombosis** – becoming curdled]
	*L	**Bolus**
lumpy	*L	**Grumus**
lung	G	**Pneumon, pleumon** [**Pneo** – to breathe]
	L	**Pulmo** [Related to **pneumon** (G)]
lust	G	**Epithymia** [**Epithymeo** – to covet, desire, long for]

M

madness	G	**Lyssa** – also, rabies (in dogs).
maiden	G	**Core**
maimed	G	**Peros** – also, helpless, disabled.
make, to	L	**Facio**
make acid, to	G	**Oxyno**
make clear, to	G	**Phaino**
make gentle, pliable, to	L	**Emollio** – also, to soften [**Mollis** – soft, tender]
make ready, to	G	**Stello**
malaria	L	**Mephitis**
male	G	**Arrhenicos**
	L	**Virilis**

mallet	G	**Sphyra**
man	G	**Aner**
	L	**Vir**
mange	G	**Alopex, alopecia**
manifest	G	**Phaneros** [**Phaino** – to shine forth, make clear]
mankind	G	**Anthropos** – also, man, slave, fellow, one.
manner	G	**Hodos** – also, course, way forward, journey, method or system.
many	G	**Polys**
	L	**Multus**
marine	G	**Thalassa**
mark	G	**Gnomon** [**Gignosco** – to know, perceive, think]
		Stigma [**Stizo** – to tattoo, mark]
	L	**Vestigium** [**Vestigo** – to track down]
marriage	G	**Gamos**
marriage bed	G	**Eune** – also, bed, lair, grave. [**Eunazo** – to lie in ambush; to put to bed; give in marriage]
marrow	G	**Myelos** – also, fatty, soft meat.
		Medulla [**Medius** – middle]
masculine	G	**Arrhenicos**
	L	**Virilis**
mass	G	**Oncos** – also, flatulent distension, volume; dignity, bombast. [**Oncoo** – to raise up, exalt, distend, be puffed up, elated]
mastic	G	**Mastiche**
masticate, to	G	**Mastichao**
matrix	*G	**Stroma**
matter	G,L	**Hyle**
	G	**Stenos**
	L	**Jejunus**
meal	L	**Prandium** [**Prandeo** – to have lunch. Related to **proen** (G) just now, lately]
measure	G	**Emmetria**
		Metron [Related to **metior** (L) – to measure]
meat	G	**Broma** [**Bibrosko** – to eat]
		Creas
meats, cooked	G	**Opson**
medicine	G	**Dynamis**

melting	G	Chysis
membrane	G	Chorion
		Hymen
		Meninx, meninges (plur.)
	L	Indusium
memory	G	Mnena, mnene [Mnaomai – to turn one's mind to, court, solicit]
meniscus	G	Meniscos [dim. of meis, mene, menos – month, lunar month, crescent moon, crescentic form]
mercury	G	Hydrargyros [Hydros – liquid, and argyros – silver]
micturate, to	G	Oureo
	L	Mingo, mictum
middle	G	Mesos (mese, meson)
	L	Medius [Related to mesos (G)]
middle plane	*L	Sagitta
midriff	G	Phren – also, the mind, wits, will.
migration	G	Metoicia [Metoicizo – to emigrate]
mild	G	Malacos [Malasso – to make soft, supple]
milk	G	Gala – also, the sap of plants.
		Pion
	L	Lac – also, the sap of plants. [Related to gala (G)]
millet seed	L	Millium
millstone	G	Myle
	L	Mola
mind	G	Noos, nous – also, heart and soul, reason, intellect.
		Phren – also, the midriff, wits, will.
		Thymos
	L	Mens (not to be confused with mensis – month)
mire	G	Pelos
mirror		Speculum – also, a copy. [Specio – to look at, behold. Related to sceptomai – to look out for, examine]
miscarriage	G	Ectrosis
	L	Abortus
misfortune	G	Ptoma [Pipto – to fall down]
mist	G	Aer

mistletoe	G	**Ixos**
	L	**Viscum**

Both words refer to the mistletoe whose berries were used as birdlime, and thus to sticky substances.

mite	G	**Acari.** A kind of mite which breeds in beeswax. [Related to **acares** – small, instantly. This comes from **a** and **keino** – to cut short, and indicates that mites are so small they cannot be subdivided]
mitigate, to	L	**Lenio** – also, to calm down. [**Lenis** – gentle, mild]
mixture	G	**Crasis**
	L	**Mixtura**
mode of life	G	**Bios**
moist	G	**Hygros** – also, soft, languid, flaccid, dainty, voluptuous.
	L	**(H)umor**
molar tooth	G	**Gomphios**
		Myle
mole (on skin)	L	**Naevus**
monkey	G	**Pithecos** – also, a dwarf.
monster	G	**Chimaira**
	*	**Ectroma** [**ec** – from, and **troma** (**trauma**) – a festering wound]
		Teras [**Terastios** – a monstrous birth]
month	G	**Mene**
	L	**Mensis**

Both are connected with the lunar month and thus with the moon.

moon	G	**Mene**
		Selene – also, month, crescentic-shaped.
	L	**Luna** – also, night, month, crescentic-shaped.
more	G	**Pleion**
	L	**Per**
morsel	G	**Psomos**
mother	L	**Mater**
motion	L	**Actus**
mound	G	**Boubon**

mouse	G	**Mys** – also, rat, jerboa, mussel, a form of whale. The same word is used for muscle (q.v.).
mouth	G	**Stoma**
	L	**Os**
		Both mean also the mouth as the organ of speech the face, the front, an entrance.
mouthwash	L	**Collutorium** [**col** – with, and **lutum** – washed. Related to **luo** (G) – to wash]
move, to	G	**Kineo** – also, to disturb, to be agitated, excited.
	L	**Curro** – associated with running a race.
		Moveo – also, to move oneself, to dislodge, to move mentally, excite.
movement	*G	**Athetos**
		Kinesis
	L	**Actus**
		Motus [**Moveo** – to move]
movement away	L	**A, ab**
mucus	G	**Blenna**
		Coryza
		Myxa
mud	G	**Pelos**
murder, to	L	**Caedo**
murmur	L	**Fremitus**
muscle	G	**Mys.** This is the same word as that for mouse (q.v.) but the reason for this is obscure.
		Sarx – also, the flesh of fruits.
muscles of upper arm	L	**Lacertus**
muscle ring	G	**Sphincter** – also a tight band.
mute	L	**Mutus** – also, inarticulate, silent.
mutilated	G	**Colobos** [**Coloboo** – to dock, curtail, mutilate]
mutually	G	**Allelon**
muzzling	G	**Phimosis** – also, silencing (by death) [**Phimos** – a muzzle, a bridle with pipes which were sounded by the horse's breath]
myopic	G	**Bathos**
myself	G,L	**Ego**

N

nail	G	Onyx
	L	Unguis
nails, hooked or ingrown	G	Gryposis [Grypoomai – to become hooked]
name	G	Onoma – also, the reputation of someone.
nape of neck	G	Lophos
narrow	G	Stenos [Stenoo – to confine, narrow. Stenosis – being restricted]
nausea	G	Nausia [Naus – a boat, ship]
nature of something	G	Physis – also, origin, natural order, appearance.
navel	G	Omphalos
	L	Umbilicus
near	G	Peri
		Plesios
	L	Juxta [Jungo – to unite, connect]
neck	G	Deire
		Trachelos
	L	Cervix
		Collum, collus
necklace	L	Monile
needle	L	Acus [Acuo – to sharpen, make pointed]
negation	G	A, an
		Cata
	L	In
nerve	*G	Neuron
nest	L	Nidus
net	G	Arkys
	L	Rete
new	G	Cainos
		Neos [Related to novus (L) – new, young]
next	G	Deuteros
night	G	Nyx
	L	Nox – also, blindness.
nipple	G	Thele
	L	Mammilla

		Papilla
nod, to	L	Nuto
noise	L	Sonus [Sono – to sound, make a noise]
none	L	Nullus
norm, normal	G	Eu
	L	Norma
nose	G	Rhis – also, snout, promontory.
	L	Nasus – also, spout,
nose bleed	G	Epistaxis
nostril	G	Mycter – also, elephant's trunk; sneer, sarcasm.
notch	L	Crena. The origin of this word is uncertain.
nourished, to be	G	Threpteos
nourishment	G	Trophe [Trepho – to rear, suckle, feed]
novel	G	Cainos
		Neos [Related to novus (L) – new, young]
nucleus	*L	Nucleus

numbers	Greek	Latin
one	mono	uni
two	di	bi
three	tri	ter
four	tetra	quadra
five	penta	quinque
six	hexa	sexa
seven	hepta	septa
eight	octo	octo
nine	ennea	novem
ten	deka	decem
eleven	endeka	undecim
twelve	dodeka	duodecim
hundred	hecto	cent
thousand	chilioi	milli

numbness	G	Narce [Narcao – to grow stiff, numb]
nurse	G	Tithene [Titheo – to tend, suckle]
nursing	L	Altrix [Alo – to nourish, feed]
nut	G	Karyon

O

obelisk	G	**Obelos**
oblique	G	**Loxos**
		Plagios – also, morally crooked. [**Plazo** – to turn aside, thwart, go astray]
oblong	G	**Thyreoeides**
obscure	L	**Occultus** [**Occulo** – to cover]
obstruct, to	G	**Phrasso**
obvious	G	**Saphes** [**Saphenizo** – to make clear]
occiput	G	**Inion**
occur sudden-ly, to	L	**Fulmino**
odour	G	**Osme.** Used for both pleasant and foul smells.
oedema	G	**Chemosis**
		Oidema
oestrous	*G	**Oistros**
offspring	G	**Blastos** [**Blastano** – to bud, sprout]
		Gone
		Gonos
		Tocos
	L	**Fetus**
		Proles
often	G	**Pollakis**
		Polys
oil	G	**Elaion** [**Elaia** – the olive tree]
	L	**Oleum** [**Olea** – the olive tree]
ointment	L	**Unguentum** [**Ungo, unguo** – to anoint]
old age	G	**Geras** [**Gerasco** – to grow old]
old man	G	**Geron** – with associations of elders, chiefs.
		Presbys – with associations of wisdom, precedence.
omentum	G	**Epiploon**
on	G	**En**
		Epi
one (single)	G	**Monos**
	L	**Unus**
one another	G	**Allelon**
oneself	G	**Ego**

	L	**Ipse**
		Sui [gen. of **se, sese** – him- or herself]
one's own	G	**Idios**
	L	**Proprius**
onrush	G	**Horme** [**Hormao** – to start, begin]
open	L	**Patens, patulus** [**Pateo** – to be or lie open]
open, to	L	**Laxo** [**Laxus** – wide, loose, relaxed]
opening	G	**Endysis** [**Endyo** – to enter, go into]
		Tresis [**Tetraino** – to pierce]
	L	**Aditus**
		Foramen [**Foro** – to bore, pierce]
		Foris [Related to **foras** – out of doors]
		Hiatus – also, open mouth, gaping after. [**Hio** – to open, gape]
		Lumen
		Meatus
open place	G	**Agora**
opposite to	G	**Anti**
		Enantios [Related to **anti** (L)]
	L	**Contra**
opposition	G	**Agon, agonos** [**Agonizomai** – to contend for a prize, struggle, fight]
		Enantios – also, contrary, against.
order	G	**Tagma** – also, fixed payment, division of soldiers, order, rank, status. [Both are from **tasso** – to be placed in order]
origin	G	**Arche**
		Genesis
		Physis – also, appearance, natural order, nature, kind.
other	G	**Heteros**
out of	G	**Ec**
outer layer	G	**Lemma**
outer tunic	L	**Indusium**
outside	G	**Ectos**
		Epi
		Exo
		Extra

ovaries	G	Didymoi
	L	Ova
over	G	Dia
		Hyper
	L	Super
		Supra
ox	G	Bous

P

pain	*G	Agreo
		Algos [Algeo – to feel, suffer pain]
		Odyne [Odynao – to feel, suffer pain]
		Ponos [Penomai – to toil, work hard, be poor]
	L	Dolor [Doleo – to suffer pain]
palate	G	Ouranos, ouraniscos (gen.) – a vaulted ceiling, a tent and similarly shaped things; the heavens, sky, universe.
pale	G	Ochros
	L	Pallidus [Palleo – to be pale]
palisade	L	Vallum [Vallus – a stake]
palm (hand)	G	Thenar – also, flat of the foot.
palpation	G	Ps>elaphesis [Pselaphao – to feel, grope for; touch, handle, examine]
panic	G	Phobos [Phebomai – to flee in terror, be put to flight]
panting	G	Asthma [Asthmazo – to pant, gasp for breath]
paradoxical	G	Atopos – also, out of place, unnatural. [a – not and topos, a place, position]
paralysed	G	Apoplecticos [Apoplexia – madness, apoplexy]
paralysis	G	Paresis
parchment	G	Hymen
parrot	G	Psittacos
part	G	Meros – also, a share, lot, destiny.
pass, to	L	Meo
passage	G	Poros
	L	Meatus [Meo – to go, pass]
passion	G	Oistros [Oistresis – mad passion]

paste	G	**Magma**
patch clothes, to	L	**Sarcio** [**Sartum** – repaired, mended]
pathway	G	**Hodos** – also, course, way forward, journey.
paunch	G	**Ascos**
pea	L	**Pisum**
pear	L	**Pirum**
peel	G	**Lemma**
	L	**Putamen** [**Puto** – to cleanse, prune, reckon up]
penetrating	G	**Embolos**
penis	G	**Peos**
		Phallos
	L	**Mentula**
people	G	**Demos** – also, the common rural people, the popular assembly.
		Ethnos – also, clubs or societies of people, and swarms or flocks of animals.
perceive, to	L	**Sentio**
perforated	G	**Tresis, tretos** [**Tetraino** – to perforate]
perform, to	L	**Fungor** – also, to be occupied with, execute, function.
perineum	G	**Perineos**
peritoneum	G	**Epiploon**
		Peritonaios
perspiration	G	**Diaphoresis**
		Hidros
pestilence	L	**Lues** – also, a calamity. [**Luo** – to atone for, pay penalty for]
phrase	G	**Lexis** [**Lego** – to tell, recount, say]
physician	G	**Iatros** [**Iatreia** – medical treatment]
pick out, to	G	**Crino**
piece	G	**Clasma** [**Clao** – to break]
pierce, to	G	**Nysso**
		Peiro. From this word comes **diapeiresis** which is a more correct term than **diapedesis**. **Diapeiresis** means the passage of cells through blood vessel walls and has nothing to do with **pedesis**, which refers to the leaping of flames over a fire. [**Diapei-**

		ro – to drive through, to interdigitate]
		Trypao
pill	G	**Coccos** – also, the testicles; female pudenda.
pillar	G	**Cion, kion**
		Stylos
pillow	L	**Pulvinus**
pimple	G	**Papula**
		Pustula
pimpled, to be	G	**Chalazao** [**Chalaza** – a small swelling, pimple, knot]
pin	G	**Perone**
	L	**Fibula**
pine cone	G	**Conos**
pipe	G	**Solen**
		Syrinx – also, cat-call (in theatre), pores and tubes in lungs.
	L	**Fistula** – also, a kind of ulcer.
pit	L	**Fovea, foveola** (dim.)
pith		**Medulla** [**Medium** – middle]
pivot	G	**Stropheos** – also, the socket in which the gudgeon pin turned; a vertebra. [**Strepho** – to turn, rotate]
place	G	**Topos**
	L	**Locus** [**Loco** – to put, place]
place in order, to	G	**Tasso**
placed	G	**Statos**
placing	G	**Thesis** – also, a deposit (of money), pledge, situation. [**Tithemi** – to place, put]
plague	G	**Nosos** [**Nosema** – disease; **nosazo** – to be ill]
	L	**Lues** – also, a calamity. [**Luo** – to atone for, pay penalty for]
plain	G	**Leios** [**Leioo** – to make smooth]
		Saphes [**Saphenizo** – to make clear]
plant	G	**Phyton** [**Phyo** – to produce, beget, spring up, get shoots]
plaque	G	**Elasma**
		Plax
	L	**Pinguis**

please, to	L	**Placeo**
pleasing	L	**Benignus** [**Beo** – to bless, please, and **gigno** – bring forth]
pleasure	G	**Hedone** [**Hedomai** – to enjoy oneself]
pliant	G	**Streptos**
	L	**Mollis**
ploughshare	L	**Vomer**
pluck at, to	G	**Tillo**
point	G	**Acme**
		Stigma [**Stizo** – to tattoo, mark]
	L	**Acumen** – also, sharpness of wit, cunning. [**Acuo** – to sharpen, make pointed]
		Cuspis
		Punctum [**Pungo** – to prick, puncture]
poison	L	**Toxicum**
	L	**Virus**
poison, to	L	**Veneno** – also, to drug. [**Venenum** – a drug, love-potion, dye]
polish, to	G	**Aleipho** [**Aleipsis** – anointing]
poor	G	**Amblys**
		Cacos
poppy juice	G	**Mecon**
porous	G	**Poros** – also, a ferry, ford, strait, bridge. [Possibly related to **peiro** – to pierce or **perao** – to pass through, penetrate]
porous stone	L	**Tofus**
porridge	G	**Athare** [**Atheroma** – a tumour containing gruel-like matter]
possess	G	**Hexis** [**Echo** – to have, hold, keep]
possess, to	G	**Echo**
position	G	**Stasis** [**Istemi** – to stand, set up, cause]
		Topos
pouch	*L	**Bursa**
pour, to	G	**Cheo**
		Rheo
	L	**Fundo**
poverty	G	**Penia** [**Peneo** – to be poor]
power	G	**Cratos** [**Cratyno** – to strengthen, confirm, govern]

		Dynamis
		Sthenos [**Stheno** – to have strength, power, be might]
	L	**Vis**
prattle, to	G	**Laleo** [**Lalos** – talkative, loquacious]
predisposition	G	**Catarxis**
pregnancy	G	**Cyesis** [**Cyeo** – to conceive]
pregnant	L	**Gravidus** [Related to **gravis** and **barys** (G) – heavy]
		Pregnans [**Prae** – before and (g)**natans**, from (g)**nascor**. – born. Related to **gigno** – to give birth]
prematurely born	L	**Abortus**
prepuce	G	**Posthe** – also, the penis, a stye on the eye.
preputial secretion	G	**Smemma, smegma**
press, to	G	**Piezo** [**Piesis** – compression, squeezing]
		Thlibo
	L	**Trudo**
pressure	G	**Thlipsis** – also, crushing, oppression, castration. [**Thlibo** – to press]
prick, to	G	**Centeo** – also, to goad, stab, spur on. [**Centesis** – pricking, mosaic]
		Peiro
prickle	G	**Acantha**
produce, to	G	**Phyo** [**Physis** – origin, nature]
	L	**Facio**
production	G	**Poiesis** [**Poieo** – to make, produce, create, cause, procure]
progeny	G	**Gone**
		Gonos
prominence	L	**Umbo**
prominent	G	**Basilicos**; really kingly, royal, choice. [**Basileus** – king, **basileia** – queen]
promote growth, to	G	**Trepho** – also, to thicken a liquid, to be reared (especially during the first five years), cherish, nourish, educate.
prone	L	**Pronus**
prong	G	**Odous**

proper	G	Deon
		Emmetria
property	G	Symptoma
protruberance	L	Furunculus [This could be related to furero – to ravage, or ferveo – to be hot]
		Torus – also, a knot, bed, mattress, couch.
provoke	G	Erithizo – also, to rouse to anger [Erithismos – irritation, stimulation, provocation]
puberty	G	Tragos
pubes, pubic region	G	Epision, sometimes wrongly spelt episeion.
		Hebe – the period before adulthood for youths; youthful spirits [Hebao – to have attained puberty, to be young and vigorous]
	L	Pubes
pull, to	G	Tillo
	L	Traho
		Vello
pulse	G	Sphygmos
pulverisation	L	Tritura [Tero – to rub, grind, thresh]
puncture, to	*G	Centeo
pupil, of eye	G	Core
pupil dilation	G	Mydriasis
purgation	G	Catharsis [Cathairo – to purge, cleanse]
purple	G	Porphyra
	L	Purpura
purulent	L	Purulentus
pus	G	Pyon [Pyoo – to suppurate]
	L	Pus – also, gall, venom.
push, to	L	Trudo
pustule	G	Pemphix
	L	Papula
		Pustula
putrefaction	G	Sepsis [Opposite to pepsis]
putrid	G	Sapros [Sepo – to make putrid]

Q

quake, to	G	Seio

quaking	G	**Tromos** [**Tromeo** – to tremble, shake – especially from fear]
quick	G	**Tachys, tachistos** (sup.)
quicken	L	**Celero**
quiver, to	G	**Pallo** – also, to brandish, poise, draw lots. **Tromeo**

R

rabid	G	**Lyssa** – also, madness, frenzy.
race	G	**Ethnos** – also, clubs or societies of people, and swarms or flocks of animals. **Genos** **Gone** **Gonos** **Phyle** – also, a tribe, clan, or a subdivision of these.
	L	**Genus** [**Geno, gigno** – to bring forth. Related to **genos** (G)]
radial structures	G	**Actis**
radiate, to	L	**Radior**
rag	L	**Pannus**
rainbow	G	**Iris**
range over, to	G	**Poleo** [**Polesis** – movement]
rapid	G	**Tachys, tachistos** (sup.)
	L	**Celer**
rare	G	**Manos** – also, loose, spreading. [**Manoo** – to make loose, porous] **Spanios, spanos**
rarified	L	**Rarus**
rasp	G	**Xyster**
rattling	G	**Crotos**
raw	G	**Omos**
ray	G	**Actis**
	L	**Radius**
rear	G	**Opisthen**
receive, to	L	**Recipio** [**re** – again and **capio** – to take, catch, receive]
reciprocally	G	**Allelon**

recollection	G	**Mnema, mnene** [**Mnaomai** – to turn one's mind to, court, solicit]
red	G	**Erythros**
	L	**Ruber**
reddish-brown	G	**Porphyra**
redness	G	**Erythema**
redness of the dawn	G	**Eos**
reduce, to	G	**Meioo**
reed	G	**Calamos**
refuse	L	**Faex**
relax, to	G	**Chalao** [**Chalasis** – loosening, relaxation]
	L	**Laxo**
release, to	L	**Mitto**
remedy	G	**Acesis, acos** [Both are from **aceomai** – to cure, remedy]
		Pharmacon
removal	G	**Ectome**
		Metoicia [**Metoicizo** – to emigrate]
removed	G	**Ec-** , **ex -**
		Ectome
	L	**Ablatus**
repair	L	**Sarcio** [**Sartum** – repaired, mended]
repetition	*G	**Palin**
	L	**Re-**
resist, to	L	**Calcitro**
responsibility	G	**Aitia** [**Aitios** – culpable; **aitiaomai** – to accuse]
restlessness	*	**Jactation**
restraint	L	**Frenum**
		Habena [**Habeo** – to have, hold]
		Viculum [**Vincio** – to bind]
		All three words are associated with bridle, reins and bands.
restrict, to	L	**Coarto**
retain, to	G	**Ischo**
retention	G	**Cathexis** [**Catecho** – to check, restrain, hold fast]
		Schesis [**Echo** – to have, hold]
return home, to	G	**Nosteo**

reveal, to	G	Phaino
	L	Aperio [Apertus – open; apertum – an open space]
revolution	L	Vertigo
rheum	L	Pituita
rheumatism	G	Arthron, arthriticos
rib	G	Pleuron
	L	Costa
ribbon	G	Lemniscos
		Tainia – also, bandage, fillet, strip of land.
ridge	G	Lophos
	L	Crista [Related to crinis – hair on the head]
right (correct)	G	Deon
right-hand side	G	Dexios [Opposite to aristeros – on the left-hand side]
rigidity (of joints)	G	Ankylosis [Ankyloo – to bend]
rind	G	Lemma
	L	Putamen [Puto – to cleanse, prune, reckon up]
ring	G	Cricos, circos – also, eyelet-hole, chain-link, hoop. Gyros [Gyroo – to make round]
ringing	L	Tinnitus
rinsed	L	Collutum [col – with, and (ab)lutum – to wash]
rod	G	Rhabdos
rod, small	G	Bactron, bacteria
	L	Bacillum [Dim. of baculum – a staff or stick. Related to bactron (G) – a stick or cane]
roof	L	Tectum [Tego – to cover]
room	L	Atrium – also, a house.
root	G	Rhiza
	L	Radix
rope	L	Restis
rose	G	Rhodon – also, rose-colour.
rotation	G	Dine, dinesis [Dino – to thresh by the treading of circling oxen]
	L	Turbo [Related to turba – tumult, commotion and tyrbe (G) – confusion, tumult]
rotten	G	Sapros [Sepo – to make putrid]
	L	Caries

rouge	G	**Phycos** – also, seaweed, sedge.
rough	G	**Trachys** – also, jagged, hard, shaggy.
	L	**Asper** [**Aspero** – to roughen]
round	G	**Cyclos** – also, ring, wheel, sphere.
		Gyros [**Gyroo** – to make round]
		Strongylos [**Strongyloo** – to make round]
round boss	G	**Omphalos**
row, of men	G	**Stichos**
royal	G	**Basilicos**; really kingly, important, choice. [**Basileus** – king; **basileia** – queen]
rub, to	G	**Thlibo**
		Tribo
	L	**Tero** – also, to grind, thresh. [Related to **tribo** (G)]
run, to	L	**Curro** – associated with running a race.
		Fluo
run	G	**Dromos** – also, a race, race-course, collonade [Related to **dramein** from **trecho** – to run, move quickly]
rung (of ladder)	G	**Climacter** [**Climax** – a ladder; from **clino** – to lean]

S

S-shaped	G	**Sigma**
sac	L	**Alveus**
		Bursa
		Utriculus
sacculations	*L	**Haustra**
sacrum	G	**Hieros**
	L	**Sacer, sacrum**
		In both languages, these words mean sacred or holy, yet have connexions with the lower spine. The reason for this association is obscure.
sail	L	**Velum**
saliva	G	**Sialon**
salt	G	**Hals**
salty	G	**Halismos**

same	G	Homoios
sand	G	Psammos
satiety	G	Coros
satyr	G	Satyros
sausage	G	Allas
	L	Botulus
saw, to	G	Prio
saw-toothed	L	Serratus
scabby	G	Lepros
scale	L	Squama
scaly	G	Ichthys
		Lepros
scar	G	Eschara
		Oule
	L	Cicatrix
scarce	G	Spanios, spanos
scent	G	Osme – both foul and pleasant smells. Also the sense of smell.
scirus	G	Sciros
scrape, to	G	Xeo
scraper	G	Xyster
scrapings	G	Xysme – also, particles, motes, shavings, filings.
screech, to	L	Stideo [Stidor – a creaking, grating noise]
scrofula		See *sow.*
scrotum	G	Osche
scurf	G	Pityrisma, pityriasis, pityrou
	L	Furfur
scurvy	L	Scorbutus
sea	G	Thalassa
seal (animal)	G	Phoce
seam	G	Rhaphe [Rhapto – to sew, stitch together]
sea-sickness		See *ship.*
seat	L	Sella, sedes [Sedeo – to sit]
sea-urchin	G	Echinos
second	G	Deuteros
see, to	G	Blepo
seed	G	Coccus – also, the testicles, female pudenda.
		Sperma [Speiro – to sow seed, scatter, strew]

	L	Semen
seize, to	G	Agreo
seizing	G	Lepsis – also, accepting, receiving. [Epilepsy is from epilepsia; epilambano – to seize, take hold of]
seizure	L	Ictus
seldom	G	Oligakis [Oligos – few, small]
		Spanios, spanos
self	G	Autos
		Psyche
semblance	G	Eicon – also, image, phantom.
sensation	G	Aisthesis [Aisthanomai – to perceive with the senses]
sense	G	Noos, nous – also, heart and soul, reason, intellect.
sense of pain	G	Algesis [Algeo – to feel pain, physical or mental]
separate, to	G	Aphaireo [Aphaeresis – removal, amputation, abstraction]
		Crino
		Orizo
separation	G	Crisis [Crino – to separate]
sequestered	G	Anachoresis [Anachoreo – to go back, retire, withdraw]
serous fluid	G	Ichor
serum	G	Oros
sesame seed	G	Sesame
setting, a	G	Thesis – also, deposit (of money), pledge, situation. [Tithemi – to place, put]
settle down, to	G	Hizano
sever, to	G	Temno – also, to prune, slaughter, divide.
	L	Seco – also, to amputate, castrate, divide.
severance	G	Tmesis [Temno – to sever, cut]
shadow	G	Skia
shaft	L	Manubrium [Related to manus – the hand]
shake, to	G	Pallo – also, to brandish, poise, draw lots.
		Seio
	L	Vibro
shameful	L	Pudendus [Pudeo – to be ashamed]
shape	L	Forma [Formo – to shape, form]

sharp	G	Oxys
sheath	G	Coleon
		Elytron
	L	Tunica
		Vagina
shell	G	Conche
shield-shaped	G	Thyreoeides (i.e., oblong)
shin, shin-bone	L	Crus
shine, to	G	Phaino
	L	Luceo
shining forth	G	Eclampsis
ship	G	Naus
shoot	G	Blastos [Blastano – to bud, sprout)
		Clados
short	G	Brachys
shoulder	G	Omos
shoulder blade	L	Scapula
shrinkage	*G	Airesis
shrivelled	*G	Krauros
shut, to	G	Kleio
shut, to be	G	Myo
sibling	G	Adelphos. This word was used of both brothers and sisters, although **adelphe** meant just sisters. **Adelphos** also meant colleague, kinsman and anything paired, e.g., twins. [**Delphys** – a womb]
sickle	G	Drepane [Drepo – to pluck, acquire]
	L	Falx
sickly	L	Morbidus
side of body	G	Pleuron
	L	Latus
sieve	G	Ethmos [Etheo – to sift, strain]
	L	Cribrum [Related to **cerno** – to separate, sift]
sight	G	Blepo, blepsomai (fut.) Scopeo – also, to behold, examine, consider. Opsis – also, the eye, pupil, iris. [From **opsomai**, the future tense of **horao** – to see, look, have sight. This root also is related to **opter** – one who spies out the land]

sign	G	Semeion – also, a signal, flag, watch-word, distinguishing mark. [Semeioo – to mark, diagnose, examine]
silica	L	Silex
silver	G	Argyros
simple	G	Haploos – also, frank, single, simple-minded, unmixed, pure.
simulate, to	G	Skepto [Skepsis – pretext, excuse, pretence]
simultaneously	G	Hama
sinew	G	Is, inos (gen.) Neuron (original meaning) Tenon
single	G	Haploos – also, frank, simple-minded, unmixed, pure.
sit fast, to	G	Hizano
sitting	G	Cathisis [Cathernai – to be seated, sit quiet, lie idle, reside]
skein	L	Glomus [Glomero – to make into a sphere, or round heap. Related to globus – a round ball, sphere]
skin	G	Chroma Chros Dartos Derma [Both dartos and derma are related to dero – to skin or flay animals]
	L	Bursa Corium, corius Cutis Pellis (from Latin via Italian)
skull	G	Cranion
slacken, to	G	Chalao [Chalasis – loosening, relaxation]
sleep	G	Caros [Caroo – to stun, stupefy] Hypnos [Hypnoo – to sleep, fall asleep]
	L	Somnus Sopor – also, deep sleep, the sleep of death. [Both somnus and sopor are from sopio – to put to sleep, stun]

slender	L	**Subtilis** – also, discriminating. [**Tela** – a fine web; **texo** – to weave]
slime	G	**Myxa** – also, synovial fluid. [**Myssomai** – to blow the nose]
	L	**Pituita**
		Virus
slip, to	G	**Olisthano**
	L	**Cado**
		Labor
slip forwards, to	L	**Prolabor**
slope	L	**Clivus**
slow	G	**Bradys**
	L	**Tardus**
small	G	**Micros**
		Oligos
	L	**Parvus**
smear over, to	L	**Lino** – also, to erase writing from waxen tablets.
smell	G	**Bromos**
		Osme. Used for both pleasant and foul smells.
smell, to	G	**Ozo**
	L	**Olfacio**
smell, sense of	G	**Osphresis**
smite, to	G	**Ballo**
		Copto
smoke	G	**Capnos** [**Capnizo** – to make smoke, fumigate]
smooth	G	**Leios** [**Leioo** – to make smooth]
		Lissos [**Lissoo** – to make insolvent; but: **lissomai** – to pray for, beg for]
	L	**Teres**
snail	L	**Cochlea, coclea** [Related to **cochlias** (G) – spiral or helical in shape; a screw, reel, roller]
snake	G	**Ophis**
snore, to	G	**Rhenco** [**Rhencos** – snoring]. See also *wheezing.*
snout	G	**Mycter** – also, elephant's trunk; sneer, sarcasm.
	L	**Rostrum** – also, beak (of birds).
soap	G	**Smema, smegma** [**Smao** – to cleanse with soap, or other unguent]
	L	**Sapo.** Originally from Celtic.

socket (deep)	G	Cotyle
socket (shallow)	G	Glene
soft	G	Malacos [Malasso – to make soft, supple]
		Thelys [Thelnyo – to make feminine]
	L	Mollis [Mollio – to make pliable, soft]
soften, to	L	Emollio
soften food, to	G	Pepsis [Pesso – to soften food by heat, cook]
solar plexus	*G	Epithymia
sole	G	Tarsos – also, wicker-work crate, palm (of hand), and similar flat structures.
solid	G	Stereos
sonorous	G	Lampros
soothe, to	L	Lenio – also, to calm down. [Lenis – gentle, mild; lenitas, lenitudo – gentleness, smoothness]
		Mulceo – also, to stroke gently, appease, charm.
sore	G	Helcos [Helcoo – to wound, lacerate, suppurate]
	L	Ulcus [Ulcero – to make sore. Related to helcos (G)]
soul	G	Psyche
		Thymos
sound	G	Phone – also, utterance, cry, phrase. [Phoneo – to produce sound or speech, utter cries, call]
		Phthongos [Phthengomai – to speak loud and clear, as a battle-cry; recite, tell of, celebrate an event]
	L	Sonor, sonus [Sono – to sound out, make a noise]
soup	L	Jus
sow	L	Scrofa [Related to gromphas (G) – an old sow. It is also said that the disease scrofula gives a pig-like expression of the face; scrofula is dim. of scrofa]
spasm	G	Spasmos [Spao – to cause convulsions, spasms]
		Sphacelos [Sphacelizo – to mortify, have convulsions, spasms]
	L	Subsulto
spectrum	*L	Spectrum
speech	G	Lexis [Lego – to tell, recount, say]
		Phasis – also, rumour, tidings. [Pheme – prophecy, speech]

		Phrasis [**Phrazo** – to point out, declare, advise, perceive]
spherical	G	**Strongylos** [**Strongyloo** – to make round]
spider's web	G	**Arachne** – also, a spider, sundial.
spike	G	**Acantha**
		Odous
spindle	L	**Fusus**
spine	G	**Acantha**
		Odous
spiral	G	**Helix** [**Helisso** – to round (a marker), dance round]
	L	**Cochlea, coclea** [Related to **cochlias** (G) – spiral or helical in shape; a screw, reel, roller]
spirit	G	**Psyche**
		Thymos
spit	G	**Obelos** (**odelos**), **obeliscos** – also, skewer, nail, obelisk.
spit, to	G	**Ptyo**
spleen	G	**Splen**
	L	**Lien**
splendid	G	**Lampros**
split	G	**Schisis** [**Schizo** – to split]
split, to	G	**Schizo**
	L	**Findo**
spoon	L	**Cocleare, cochleare**
spot	L	**Punctum** [**Pungo** – to prick, puncture]
spread on, to	L	**Lino** – also, to erase writing from waxen tablets.
spring	G	**Crene**
spring-water	L	**Lympha**
sprout	L	**Germen**
spur	L	**Calcar** [**Calx** – the heel]
squeeze, to	G	**Peizo** [**Piesis** – compression, squeezing]
		Thlibo
squinting	G	**Strabismos** [**Strabizo** – to squint]
stable	L	**Stabilis** [**Sto** – to stand. Related to **histemi** (G) – to stand]
stalk	*L	**Pediculus** – dim. of **pes**; **pedicellus** is dim. of **pediculus**.
standard	L	**Norma**

standing	G	**Stasis, statos** [**Histemi** – to stand]
standing before	G	**Prostate** [**Prohistemi** – to set before, put in front]
star	G	**Aster, astron**
	L	**Stella** [Related to **aster** (G) – a star]
starch	G	**Amylon** – also, the finest meal, a cake made with this.
start, to	G	**Hormao**
		Stello
starving	G	**Nestis**
state	G	**Hexis, schesis** [**Echo** – to have, possess, hold, keep]
	L	**Status**
statement	G	**Phasis** – also, rumour, tidings.
stature	G	**Mecos** [Related to **macros** (G) – large]
stench	G	**Bromos**
		Mephitis
step	G	**Basis, bathmos** [**Baino** – to go, walk]
step, to	L	**Gradior**
stickiness		See *mistletoe.*
stiff, to be	G	**Ankyloo**
sting	L	**Acumen** – also, sharpness of wit, cunning. [**Acuo** – to sharpen, make pointed]
sting, to	G	**Centeo** – also, to goad, stab, spur on. [**Centesis** – pricking; mosaic]
stinging nettle	L	**Urtica** [**Uro** – to burn. Related to **eyo** (G) – to singe]
stink	G	**Bromos**
stirrup	L	**Stapes** [Originally **staffa** or **stapha**.]
stocky	G	**Pyknos** [**Pyknoo** – to pack closely, condense]
stomach	G	**Gaster**
		Stomachos
stone	G	**Lithos**
		Petros
	L	**Calx, calculus** (dim.)
		Silex
stool		**Sella, sedes** [**Sedeo** – to sit]
stooping	L	**Pronus**
stop up, to	L	**Obturo**
straight	G	**Ithys** [**Ithyo** – to press straight on]

		Orthos
	L	**Rectus** [**Rego** – to direct, govern]
straining	G	**Teinesmos** [**Teino** – to stretch, strain]
	L	**Nisus**
strange	G	**Allotrios**
		Atopos – also, paradoxical, unnatural. [**a** – not, and **topos** – a place, position]
stranger	G	**Xenos**
strength	G	**Cratos** [**Cratyno** – to strengthen, confirm, govern]
		Dynamis
		Sthenos [**Stheno** – to have strength, power, be mighty]
	L	**Vis**
stretch, to	G	**Teino**
	L	**Tendo**
stretched	G	**Tetanos** [**Teino** – to stretch, strain]
strike, to	G	**Copto**
		Plesso
	L	**Pello** – also, to impel, move, drive away.
string	G	**Chorde**
	L	**Funis, funiculus** (dim.)
stripe	L	**Linea** – also, a linen thread, a plumb-line, a boundary. [**Linum** – flax, linen]
strive towards, to	L	**Pepo** [Related to **petomai** (G) – to fly, dash, dart, and **pipto** – to fall, fall upon]
stroke	G	**Plege** [**Plesso** – to strike, smite]
	L	**Ictus**
		Pulsus
struggle	G	**Agon** [**Agonizomai** – to contend, struggle, fight]
stud	G	**Helos**
study	G	**Logos** [**Lego** – to tell, retell, recount]
stupor	G	**Typhos.** One of four types of fever; also delusion, humbug, vanity.
subsequent	L	**Posterus, posterior** (comp.)
substance	G,L	**Hyle**
	L	**Corpus**
substitute	L	**Succedaneus**

substitute, to	L	Succenturio
suffering	G	Pathos [Pascho – to suffer, to be affected]
		Ponos [Penomai – to toil, work hard, be poor]
sugar	G	Saccar, saccharon
sulfur, sulphur	G	Theion
summer	L	Aestivus
summit	G	Acros [Ace – a point; acis – something pointed, a needle]
		Hypsos [Hypsi – high]
sun	G	Helios
supplement	G	Prosthesis
support, to	G	Clino – also, to cause to incline, to recline.
		Skepto [Skepsis – pretext, excuse, pretence]
suppress, to	G	Ischo
suspender	G	Cremaster [Cremmanymi – to hang up, suspend]
suture	G	Rhaphe [Rhapto – to sew, stitch]
swallow, to	L	Glutio
sweat	G	Hidros [Hidroo – to sweat, perspire]
	L	Sudor [Sudo – to sweat, perspire]
sweating	G	Diaphoresis – also, plundering, evaporation, exhaustion. [Diaphoreo – to dissipate, disperse]
sweet	G	Glycys
sweetness	G	Gleucos
swell, to	G	Bryo
		Plethyo
	L	Tumeo; tumesco
swelling	G	Cele, kele – also, a hernia, a camel's hump.
		Ganglion
		Kyma [Kyo – to be pregnant]
		Oidema [Oideo – to swell]
		Phyma [Phyo – to produce, grow, create]
	L	Bulla
		Torus – also, a knot, bed, mattress, couch.
		Tuber [Tumeo – to be swollen]
swim, to	L	Nato [No – to swim; related to neo (G) – to swim]
sword	G	Xiphos
		Ensis
symptom	G	Semeion – also, a signal, flag, watch-word, distin-

guishing mark. [**Semeioo** – to mark, diagnose, examine]

Symptoma

synovial fluid   G   **Sialon**

T

tail	G	**Cercos**
	L	**Cauda**
take care of, to	G	**Comizo** – also, to attend to, preserve, acquire, extract, remove.
take up, to	L	**Suscipio**
talus	G	**Astragalos**
tape-worm	G	**Tainia** – also, ribbon, bandage, fillet.
tardy	G	**Bradys**
	L	**Tardus**
taste	G	**Geuma** [**Geuo** – to give a taste of]
	L	**Gustatus** [**Gusto** – to taste, partake of]
tattoo	G	**Stigma** [**Stizo** – to tattoo, mark]
taut	G	**Tetanos** [**Teino** – to stretch, strain]
teach, to	G	**Paideuo**
tear (drop)	G	**Dacryon** [**Dacryo** – to weep]
		Epiphora [**Epiphortizo** – to overload]
	L	**Lacrima** [**Lacrimo** – to shed tears, weep]
tear (rent)	G	**Rhexis** [**Rhegnymi** – to burst asunder]
		Spadon [**Spao** – to draw (a sword, breath), pluck out, cause convulsions, tear apart]
tear. to	G	**Eryo**
		Spao
	L	**Lacero** – also, to lame, mutilate.
teat	G	**Thele**
teem with, to	G	**Bryo**
temple (of the head)	G	**Crotaphos** [**Crotaphizo** – to hit on the temple]
	L	**Tempus** – also, a period of time. [Related to **temno, temenos** (G) – to divide; separated precinct]
tender	L	**Mollis** [**Mollio** – to make pliable, soft]
tendon	G	**Neuron** (original meaning)

		Tenon
tendril (of vine)	L	**Pampinus**
tension	G	**Tonos** [**Teino** – to stretch]
tent	L	**Tentorium** [**Tendo** – to stretch, spread, extend]
terror	G	**Phobos** [**Phebomai** – to flee in terror, be put to flight]
testis	G	**Didymos, didymoi** (plur.) **Orchis, orcheis** (plur.) – also, ovary, olive.
thick	G	**Pachys** [**Pachyno** – to fatten, make gross, coarsen] **Pyknos** [**Pyknoo** – to pack closely, condense]
thigh	G	**Meros** – also, thigh-bone.
thirst	G	**Dipsa** [**Dipsakos** – a disease with excessive thirst, diabetes]
thorn	G	**Acantha**
thought	G	**Gnome** – also, intelligence, inclination, verdict. **Logos** [**Lego** – to tell, retell, recount] **Noema, noesis** [**Noeo** – to perceive, apprehend]
thread	G	**Byssos** **Mitos** – also, Ariadne's thread of destiny. **Nema** – also, silk sutures. [**Neo** – to spin]
	L	**Filum**
threefold	L	**Trigeminus**
three months	L	**Trimester**
threshing (corn)	L	**Tritura** [**Tero** – to rub, grind]
threshold	G	**Bathmos** [**Baino** – to go, walk]
	L	**Limen inferum**
throat	G	**Deire** **Pharynx** **Stomachos** **Trachelos**
	L	**Faux** **Guttur** **Jugulum.** Related to the neck, on which a yoke rested. [**Jungo** and **zeugnymi** (G) – to unite, join, yoke together]
throb, to	G	**Pedao**
throng	G	**Ochlos**
through	G	**Dia**

	L	Per
throw	G	Bole [Ballo – to throw]
throw, to	G	Ballo
	L	Jacio – also, to throw away, scatter, fling.
thrush (disease)	G	Aphtha, aphthai (plur.)
thrust	G	Osme, osmos [Otheo – to push, thrust]
tie, to	L	Ligo [Ligamen – a string, binding]
tissue	G	Enchyma
	*	Histos
toad	G	Phryne
together (with)	G	Syn
	L	Cum
tomb	G	Thece
tongue	G	Glossa
	L	Lingua – also, speech, language.
tonsil	G	Amygdale – also, almond.
tooth	G	Odous
	L	Dens
toothless	L	Edentulus
top	G	Acron [Ace – a point; acis – something pointed, a needle]
		Hypsos [Hypsi – high]
torpor	G	Narce [Narcao – to grow stiff, numb]
touch	G	Haphe [Haptomai – to fasten, bind, take hold of]
		Pselaphesis [Pselaphao – to feel, grope for, handle, examine]
touch, to	G	Hapto
	L	Palpo, palpor – also, to coax, wheedle, flatter.
		Tango – also, to reach, strike, steal.
tough	L	Durus – also, uncouth, austere, severe.
towards	G,L	Ad
	L	Versus, versum
transformation	G	Allaxis
treat medically, to	G	Therapeuo [Therapon – a male attendant; therapaina – a female slave]
tree	G	Dendron, dendreon
tremble, to	L	Vibro
trembling	G	Tromos [Tromeo – to tremble, especially from fear]

trial	G	**Crisis** [**Crino** – to separate]
trifle	L	**Hilum**
triplets	L	**Trigeminus**
trough	G	**Pyelos** – also, bathing tub, sarcophagus, infundibulum of the brain.
trumpet	G	**Salpinx**
trumpeter	L	**Bucinator** [**Bucina** – a bent trumpet; **tuba** – a straight trumpet]
truncated	G	**Colobos** [**Coloboo** – to dock, curtail, mutilate]
trunk	G	**Cormos** [**Ceiro** – to cut short, crop]
tube	L	**Fistula** – also, a kind of ulcer.
tumour	G	**Cele, kele** – also, a hernia, swelling, camel's hump. **-oma**, only as a suffix.
		Oncos – also, flatulent distension, volume; dignity, bombast. [**Oncoo** – to raise up, exalt, distend, be puffed up, elated]
		Phyma [**Phyo** – to produce, create, grow]
tunic	G	**Ependyma**
	L	**Indusium.** Probably an outer garment. **Tunica.** A woollen shirt or tunic worn by both men and women.
turn, to	G	**Campto**
		Trepo
	L	**Volvo**
turning	L	**Vertigo** [**Verto** – to turn round]
twice	G	**Dis**
twilight	G	**Knephas**
twins	G	**Didymoi**
	L	**Gemini** [**Gemino** – to double]
twisted	G	**Scolios**
		Speira – also, coils, circular mouldings, a kind of cake.
		Streptos
	L	**Tortum** [**Torqueo** – to twist, wrench]
twitch, to	L	**Vello**
twofold	G	**Dis, dicha**
type	G	**Eidos** [**Eido** – to see, perceive]

U

ulcer	G	**Carcinos**
		Helos [**Helcosis** – ulceration; **helcoo** – to wound, ulcerate]
	L	**Ulcus** [Related to **helcos** (G)]
ulna	G	**Olene**. See *arm, lower.*
		Pechys. See *arm, lower.*
uncleanliness	G	**Mysos**
under	G	**Hypo** – also, below, beneath.
	L	**Infra**, from **inferus**.
		Sub
understanding	G	**Noema** [**Noeo** – to perceive, apprehend]
understood	G	**Gnotos**
unending	G	**Ateles** [**a** – not, and **telos** – end]
unequal, uneven	G	**Scelenos** – also rough, oblique.
	L	**Impar** – also, odd (numbers), unlike. [**im** – not, and **par** – alike]
unguent	G	**Magma**
		Smema, smegma [**Smao** – to cleanse with soap or other unguent]
union	G	**Syzygia** – also, copulation, conjunctions in pairs, conjugations. [**Syzeugnymi** – to yoke together; **zeugos** – yoke, a pair of animals yoked together]
unitary	G	**Monas**
unite, to	G	**Arthroo** [**Arthron** – a joint; **arthrosis** – a connexion or articulation; **arthriticos** – gout, arthritis]
united	G	**Syn**
unstable	L	**Labor**
unusual	G	**Heteros** – strictly, one of two.
upon	G	**Ana**
upright	G	**Orthos**
urachus	G	**Ourachos** – also, apex of the heart, outer ends of the eyebrows, point of a drill.
urine	G	**Ouron**
urinate, to	G	**Oureo**
	L	**Mingo**
useable, useful	G	**Chrestos** – also, good, pleasant, effective, kindly.

uterus	G	**Delphys**
		Hystera
		Metra – also, the cervix of the uterus, core, source, origin.
utterance	G	**Phasis** – also, rumour, tidings. [**Pheme** – prophecy, speech]
uvula	G	**Cion, kion**
		Staphyle – a bunch of grapes, associated with the uvula because it was thought to look like a grape when swollen and inflamed.

V

vagina	G	**Colpos**
vapour	G	**Capnos** [**Capnizo** – to make smoke, fumigate]
	L	**Mephitis**
varicose vein	G	**Cirsos**
	L	**Varix**
variegated	L	**Varius** [**Vario** – to vary, diversify]
vault	G	**Ouranos, ouraniscos** – a vaulted ceiling, a tent and similarly shaped things: roof of the mouth, the palate.
	L	**Fornix**
vein	G	**Phleps** – originally either artery or vein. See *blood vessel.*
venereal	L	**Venereus, Venerius.** Since this word is derived from the name Venus, the godess of love, it could begin with a capital letter.
vertebra	G	**Sphondylos.** This word became corrupted later to **spondylos.** Also used for the drums of stone used in columns, a pebble used in voting, a roller.
vertex	G	**Obelos, odelos.** (Referring to the end of the spit, skewer, or obelisk.)
vesicle	G	**Pemphis, pemphigos** (gen.) See also *bubble.*
		Physa [**Physao** – to blow, distend, be puffed up]
vessel	G	**Angeion** – also, bucket, sack, coffin.
	L	**Vas, vasculum** (dim.)
vibrate, to	G	**Pallo** – also, to brandish, poise, draw lots.

	L	Vibro
victuals	G	Opson
vigorous	L	Vegetus [Vegeo – to quicken, liven up, excite]
visible	G	Phaneros [Phaino – to shine forth, make clear]
visitor	G	Xenos
voice	G	Phone – also, utterance, cry, phrase. [Phoneo – to produce sound or speech, utter cries, call]
void	G	Cenos, kenos [Kenoo – to empty]
	L	Vacuus – also, exempt, lacking something.
volatile	G	Ptenos [Petomai – to fly]
vomiting	G	Emesis [Emeo – to vomit]
vulva	G	Epision, epeision

W

walk, to	G	Baino
	L	Gradior
walk about, to	L	Ambulo – also, to walk to and fro, to go for a walk, to travel.
wall	G	Teichos
	L	Paries – strictly, the wall of a house.
		Saeptum [Saepio – to surround, confine]
		Vallum [Vallus – a stake]
wandering	G	Aleteia [Aleteuo – to wander, roam; especially of beggars]
	L	Vagus – also, roaming, inconstant, fickle, diffuse.
wanting, to be	G	Eremos [Eremia – a desert]
		Penia [Peneo – to be poor]
		Spanis, spanios, spanos [Spanizo – to be scarce, in want]
ward off, to	G	Alexo
		Arceo – also, to succour, suffice.
wart	G	Sycon [Sycea – the fig tree Ficus carica]
	L	Verruca
wash, to	L	Luo
wash away, to	L	Abluo
waste	*G	Spodos

wasted, to be	G	**Triphthesomai** [**Tribo** – to rub, wear out, waste, ravage]
wasting away	G	**Phthisis** [**Phthio** – to wane, decay, pine, perish]
	L	**Tabes** – also, decay, disease, pestilence. [**Tabeo** – to waste away. Related to **teko** (G) – to waste, pine away]
water	G	**Hydor**
	L	**Lympha**
watery vesicle	G	**Hydatis** [**Hydor** – water]
wave	G	**Kyma** – also, swell of the seas. [**Kyo** – to be pregnant, swollen]
wax, waxen	L	**Cera, cereus** [Related to **keros** (G) – beeswax, taper wax]
way	G	**Hodos** – also, course, way forward, journey, method or system.
		Tropos
wear (out), to	G	**Tribo**
	L	**Tero** – also, to grind, thresh. [Related to **tribo** (G)]
weariness		**Copos**
weaving	G	**Histos**
web	G	**Arachne** – also, a spider, sundial.
		Histos
		Hyphe
	L	**Tela** [**Texo** – to weave]
wedge	G	**Embolos**
		Sphen
	L	**Cuneus** [**Cuneo** – to shape like a wedge]
weight	G	**Baros** – also, torpor, influence, dignity.
well (fit)	G	**Eu**
well (spring)	G	**Crene**
well-being	G	**Euphoria**
wet	G	**Hygros**
	L	**(H)umor**
wheezing	G	**Rhochmos**, later **rhonchos** [**Rhocho** – to wheeze]
whirlpool	L	**Vertex** [**Verto** – to turn round]
white	G	**Leucos, leukos**
	L	**Albus**

Candidus – also, glistening, lucid, honest, happy. [**Candeo** – to glitter, shine]

whole	G	**Holos**
whorl	G	**Helix** [**Helisso** – to round (a marker), dance round]
	L	**Vertex** [**Verto** – to turn round]
wide	G	**Eurys** – also, broad, far-reaching, spread wide.
widen, to	G	**Euryno**
	L	**Laxo**
wife	G	**Gyne** – also, female, mistress, lady.
will	G	**Boule** – also, counsel, decree. [**Bouleuo** – to take counsel, deliberate]
will, to	L	**Volo**
wind	G	**Physa** [**Physao** – to blow, distend, be puffed up]
		Pneuma
windpipe	G	**Bronchos**
		Larynx
		Pharynx
	L	**Guttur**
window	L	**Fenestra**
wine-skin	G	**Ascos**
wing	G	**Pteryx** – also, fins of fish, seals, paddle blade, shoulder-blade.
	L	**Ala**
wink, to	L	**Nicto**
withdrawal	G	**Metachoresis** [**Metachoreo** – to go elsewhere, migrate]
withered	L	**Flaccus, flaccidus**
within	G	**Endon, entos**
		En
	L	**In**
		Intra
		Intus [Related to **entos** (G)]
witness	G	**Gnomon** [**Gignosco** – to know, perceive, think]
wolf	G	**Lycos** – also, various animals, and hook-shaped things.
	L	**Lupus** – also, a fish, a hook. [Related to **lycos** (G)]
woman	G	**Gyne** – also, female, mistress, wife.
		Nymphe

wool	G	**Mallos** – also, a tress of (men's) hair.
		Pilos – felt used inside shoes and helmets.
word	G	**Lexis** [**Lego** – to tell, recount, say]
work	G	**Ergon** [**Ergozomai** – to labour, work at]
world	G	**Chthon**
worm	G	**Ascaris** – also, the larva of the mosquito.
		Helmins, helminthos (gen.)
		Scolex – also, earthworm, larvae.
	L	**Lumbricus**
		Tinea
		Vermis [Related to **verto** – to turn round]
wound	G	**Helcos** [**Helcoo** – to wound]
		Trauma [**Traumizo** – to wound]
		Trosis [**Titrosko (troo)** – to wound, injure, kill]
	L	**Vulnus**
wound together	G	**Speira** – also, coils, circular mouldings, a kind of cake.
woven	G	**Hyphe**
wrinkle	G	**Rhytis** [Related to **rhysis** – flow, and **rheo** – to flow]
wrist	G	**Carpos**
written	G	**Gramme**

Y

yarn	G	**Nema** – also, silk sutures. [**Neo** – to spin]
yawn, to	L	**Oscito** [**Os** – mouth, and **cieo** – to move. Related to **kineo** (G) – to move]
yellow	G	**Xanthos**
	L	**Flavus** [Related to **flagro** and **phlego** (G) – to burn]
		Luteus. From the colour of the saffron plant, *Lutum*.
yellowish	G	**Cirrros**. Usually mistakenly spelt **cirrhos**.
		Ochros
yeast	G	**Zyme** [Related to **zo** – to live, quicken]
yield, to	G	**Chalao** [**Chalasis** – loosening, relaxation]

yoke	G	**Zygon** – also, a balance beam, yard-arm.
	L	**Jugum** [**Jungo** – to yoke together, unite]
yoke (egg)	G	**Lecithos**
young	G	**Neos** [Related to **novus** (L) – new, young]
youth	G	**Hebe** [**Hebao** – to be young and vigorous]

Z

| zeal | G | **Zelos** [**Zeloo** – to be jealous, envy; also to emulate, praise] |